# CUSTOMIZE
# YOURSELF

# CUSTOMIZE YOURSELF: NUTRITION

## AND WHAT I LEARNED FROM

## MY 110 YEAR OLD MOTHER

# CHUCK ROSE

**BRIELLE BOOKS**
**NEW JERSEY**

Brielle Books. Cover design by Chuck Rose. customizeyourself.org

ISBN 978-7372827-0-9 (paperback)
ISBN 978-7372827-1-6 (eBook)

*This book is dedicated to my mother, Edith Rose
who sang* YOU ARE MY SUNSHINE *to me when I was a small
child until I was delirious with laughter.*

# Contents

## Part II: *Plants And More Plants*

# Introduction

## The Journey

How do you blaze a path to a leaner, healthier, happier, less stressful, more vital, longer life?

Do you follow someone's else's route, or is it better to create your own?

Where do you start?

I started in Maplewood, New Jersey, raised by a mother who had already acquired a few skills bringing up my sister and brother, beginning 11 and 8 years before I arrived. And well before that, my mother was assigned various chores and responsibilities by my grandmother to look after her 7 siblings. Surviving the 1918 pandemic was an early episode in my family's history. With only a sweater to keep her warm, Mom was sent off to Miss Watson's third grade class at The Morton Street School in Newark with a little bag of camphor tied around her neck. I guess it worked.

Throw in the Great Depression, 2 World Wars, a 68 year marriage, and Mom always had more on her mind than TV or Tik Tok.

The subtitle of CUSTOMIZE YOURSELF is, *And What I Learned From My 110 Year Old Mother.* Edith Rose is a terrific example of a life well-lived. She is not only an inspiration to our whole family, but also to just about everyone who meets her. Every day, someone asks my mother, *How do you do it?* meaning, for the most part, *How do I get to live a long life?*

My mother has heard this question so many times, she dreads it. I think part of her frustration is that there is no easy answer. Much of my motivation for writing this book is to follow up here, and aim readers towards some new, useful and sustainable practices, techniques and discoveries to advance nutrition, fitness, mindbody connection and longevity.

At the same time, we're keeping an eye on Dr. Nir Barzilai, founding director of the Institute for Aging Research at Albert Einstein College of Medicine, and one of the leading pioneers in longevity research. Over the past 20 years, Dr. Barzilai's associates have visited me, my mother and members of our family to take blood samples and keep an eye on us. We hope that our pesky genes will eventually reveal some exportable tools for the advancement of longevity therapies. You can follow Dr. Barzilai's progress in AGE LATER, published by St. Martin's Press, 2020. Fascinating science. Stay tuned.

When I was growing up, doing everything to excess, my mother would occasionally slip in the one piece of advice that helped me survive and eventually prosper. She said, *The key is moderation.* The idea of moderation had little appeal to a kid with boundless energy, a barely-formed, ping-pong consciousness of curiosity and skepticism, and an unlimited supply of foolish behavior, but eventually it did sink in. I'm still driven by curiosity and skepticism, but luckily I've somehow reduced my output of foolish behavior. Or at least I've become less aware of my current foolish behavior. I'll take what I can get. In my mother's eyes, I will always be the kid who kicked a football through the neighbor's window, swore he'd never do it again, then somehow managed to do it again.

And now, my mother's journey continues into her 111th year. Amazing! Her guidance, inspiration, planning, managing, cooking, raising and caring gave me an excellent start to my own odyssey. I also discovered along the way that everything she so lovingly provided did not create a perfect itinerary, only because of a basic fact of life. Everyone in the whole world is *unique*, and everyone needs a *customized* plan.

Outside of your household cocoon, a blizzard of ideas about nutrition, physical and mental health, and the truth about all things, appears, multiplies, divides, and reveals endless choices and disagreements. Follow the news, pay attention in school, read all you can, and on any day, at any moment, the collected wisdom about everything is subject to radical change with the announcement of a new discovery or the explosion of an old myth. This process continues to accelerate, and it may soon be impossible to keep up.

To complicate matters, all of this has to be separated from the massive anti-science deluge of false and misleading information, propaganda and conspiracy theories now flooding old and new media. The designers and owners of social media companies have lost control of their algorithmic beasts. The effect is that many people have begun to believe that everything is a lie, and truth no longer exists. This serves the purposes of the purveyors of such garbage. As their influence grows, so does their incentive to dial up the load. The more poison they inject into their paranoia feedback loop, the more power and profit they attain. Such negativity opposes the advancement of science and knowledge in general, and improvements in mental and physical health in particular.

What to do? In the long run, it's the burden of everyone else to find ways to reverse the breakdown of shared reality, and rebuild trust. Fifty years ago, John Lennon pleaded, *Give peace a chance.* Maybe now, we can sing, *Give science a chance.* Or, G*ive reality a chance.* Promoting health and fitness is not a political act. It's a challenge to be sure. A living, growing, evolving challenge. Everything is subject to change. Everything I've learned, all that I've experienced, every single one of the several thousand books, articles, studies and stories that helped me to write what you have before you, is subject to change, amendment, correction, amplification, soaring enlightenment or crashing into a that's-so-silly-how-did-we-ever-believe-that brick wall.

All I ask of you is to join me for the ride. You don't need a long scarf or a rakish hat, but if that does the trick, go for it! Just watch out that your scarf doesn't land in the spaghetti, or get stuck in the spokes of your speeding vehicle. You'll be encouraged to consider, experiment, accept, reject, refine, enjoy and evolve as you CUSTOMIZE YOURSELF!

# Weight Management

After clearing the pandemic hurdle, an enormous health challenge for the United States is to gain mastery over weight management.

The obesity statistics in America are staggering. An extensive study completed by the Centers for Disease Control and Prevention (CDC) in 2018 found that the prevalence of obesity in the United States was 42.4%. Combine the obese numbers with those who are overweight, and the total is 72%.[1] And, it is predicted that the situation will get much worse. A study published in THE NEW ENGLAND JOURNAL OF MEDICINE projects that by 2030, nearly half the adults in America will be obese, and in as many 29 states, the prevalence of obesity will be more than 50%, with several near 60%.[2]

In 2020, scientists at the University of North Carolina at Chapel Hill combined data from 75 studies containing the records of 399,000 COVID-19 patients, and found that people with obesity were 113% more likely than people of healthy weight to wind up in the hospital, 74% more likely to land in an ICU, and 48% more likely to die.[3]

---

[1] "Obesity is a common, serious, and costly disease," Centers for Disease Control and Prevention, Last reviewed: June 29, 2020.
https://www.cdc.gov/obesity/data/adult.html

[2] Zachary Ward, lead author, "Projected U.S. State-Level Prevalence of Adult Obesity and Severe Obesity," THE NEW ENGLAND JOURNAL OF MEDICINE, Dec. 19, 2019.
https://www.nejm.org/doi/pdf/10.1056/NEJMsa1909301?articleTools=true

[3] Meredith Wadman, "Why COVID-19 is more deadly in people with obesity-even if they're young," SCIENCE, Sept. 8, 2020.
https://www.sciencemag.org/news/2020/09/why-covid-19-more-deadly-people-obesity-even-if-theyre-young

Snack food sales have skyrocketed because of COVID-19, and it's predicted that the trend will continue.[4]

The 'quarantine 15' will not magically disappear with a vaccine.

The average American woman today weighs more than the average 1960's man. The weight for men in 1960 averaged 166 pounds, now it's over 198 pounds. Women weighed an average of 140 pounds in 1960, now their average is over 170 pounds.[5]

Another study, also from the University of North Carolina, found that only 12% of American adults are metabolically healthy. Collecting data from 8,721 people, metabolic health was calculated on the basis of having optimal levels of 5 factors: blood glucose, triglycerides, high-density lipoprotein (HDL), blood pressure and waist circumference, without the need for medications.[6] Simply put, 88% of American adults are not meeting guidelines for cardiovascular risk factors.

---

[4] Brooke DiPalma, "COVID-19 eating created a run on snack foods in 2020, and the trend isn't done yet," YAHOO!FINANCE, Dec. 31, 2020. https://finance.yahoo.com/news/consumers-snacking-habits-increase-in-2020-prompting-innovation-return-of-90-s-favorites-135804044.html

[5] Cheryl Fryar, lead author, "Mean Body Weight, Height, Waist Circumference, and Body Mass Index Among Adults: United State, 1999-2000 Through 2015-2016," NATIONAL HEALTH STATISTICS REPORTS, Number 122, Dec. 20, 2018. https://www.cdc.gov/nchs/data/nhsr/nhsr122-508.pdf

[6] Joana Araujo, Jianwen Cai, June Stevens, "Prevalence of Optimal Metabolic Health in American Adults: National Health and Nutrition Examination Survey 2009-2016," METABOLIC SYNDROME AND RELATED DISORDERS, Vol. 17, No. 1. Published online Feb. 8, 2019. https://www.liebertpub.com/doi/10.1089/met.2018.0105

Unhealthy lifestyles and obesity are also increasing threats to national security. From 2016 to 2018, it was calculated that 71% of young people between the ages of 17 and 24 would not qualify military service, with obesity disqualifying 31% of them. This has been named as a major factor in U.S. armed forces falling short of recruitment goals.[7]

Both physical exercise and sensible diet are critical to maintain healthy, desired body weight as well as to lose weight and maintain successful weight loss. To gain weight, you consume more calories than you burn. To lose weight, you burn more calories than you consume.

It's a simple equation. You only have to abide by it to control your weight. Don't let your weight control you. You're in charge of customizing yourself.

CUSTOMIZING YOURSELF: FITNESS takes the deep plunge into how to evolve your physical activity and integrate it with your nutrition. I hope you will read it. For now, note that to maintain weight, the CDC has a general guideline of 150 minutes per week of moderate-intensity aerobic activity, suggesting 30 minutes a day, five days a week.[8] This will certainly vary from person to person. If

---

[7] Heather Maxey, Sandra Bishop-Josef, Ben Goodman, "Unhealthy and Unprepared," Council For A Strong America, Oct. 2018.
https://strongnation.s3.amazonaws.com/documents/484/389765e0-2500-49a2-9a67-5c4a090a215b.pdf?1539616379&inline;%20filename=%22Unhealthy%20and%20Unprepared%20report.pdf%22

[8] "Benefits of Physical Activity," Centers for Disease Control and Prevention, Last reviewed: Dec. 2, 2020.
https://www.cdc.gov/physicalactivity/basics/pa-health/index.htm

you're new to exercise, just get out and walk. It's safe and simple, requires no equipment or training, and you can accrue maximum benefits with a minimum of effort. You can start out at 5 or 10 minutes, add a few minutes each day, and you're up to 30 minutes per walk in a week or two. It's easy and rewarding to become an (almost) overnight walking expert!

If you're an absolute couch potato or light on exercise, 150 minutes per week is a good first goal. Get there, and when you do, mark your on calendar 6 months later, "150 MINUTES." Throw a party for yourself, then think about adding another day of exercise, or another 30 minutes, or increase your pace to burn more calories and get stronger.

As you progress, I'd certainly encourage exceeding 150 minutes a week by a good margin. I think it's an absolute minimum because if you do less, your health risks increase, and the length and quality of your life decrease. After decades of customizing, I have found that 60 to 90 minutes a day, 7 days a week, is my sweet spot. You can certainly do more, but unless you're training for a long distance or long duration event, it's not necessary.

Taking the long view, a 15 year study of 4,995 men and women found that an average American gains 2.2 pounds per year during middle age, but people who walk gain much less than those who do not. Walking benefits were greatest among the heaviest participants. A 160 pound person walking 35 minutes a day trimmed about 18 pounds over the 15 year stretch.[9]

---

[9] 'Walking: Your steps to health, HARVARD MEN'S HEALTH WATCH, Updated: Oct. 13, 2020. https://www.health.harvard.edu/staying-healthy/walking-your-steps-to-health

## Too Many Diets

Dieting is a gigantic industry. Those who have seized upon the newest, most popular diet every year have been directed, redirected and misdirected at regular intervals. At any given moment, according to the "experts," butter is bad/margarine is good, no, margarine is bad/butter is good, no, butter is bad/olive oil is good, no, wait a minute, now you can have both butter *and* olive oil, but margarine is still definitely bad. We can at least agree on that, right? Maybe. Most recent studies recommend that you replace butter with extra virgin olive oil.[10] What do the baby boomers who consumed 20 years worth of margarine do about it now? And what about eggs? Once deemed killers, now they're touted as saviors. You better stay tuned, because pretty soon we'll have some new information on that subject too.

More and more new diets are being touted, and plenty of old diets are being revived. How do you know who's got it right? Who's got it wrong? There are countless conflicts and contradictions among all these diets. How do you figure out what will work for you? Eating comes first. Everyone has to eat. Everyone likes to eat. Many people

---

[10] Sandee LaMotte, "Using olive oil instead of these foods could add years to the life of your heart, study says," CNN, Mar. 5, 2020. https://www.cnn.com/2020/03/05/health/olive-oil-heart-health-wellness/index.html

live to eat. Better that you eat to live. Or find a way to do both. The nutritional goals of CUSTOMIZE YOURSELF are to rationally improve your diet, increase enjoyment, and make yourself a leaner, healthier, better functioning person. It's a logical process of positive change. Roll with it. Have fun with it. Anyone can do it. I've been doing it for years.

If you've been exhausted by, or skeptical of the innumerable diets and self-help tomes proclaiming their veracity and necessity, you are not alone. Most require a radical change of habits which are often difficult to achieve and miserable to maintain. Any new dietary or physical regimen can be a shock to the system and possibly even be dangerous. Diets that that restrict or eliminate healthy foods can cause deficiencies, stomach upset, constipation, fatigue, malaise, bad breath, general agony and plenty of other problems. If you begin eating 10 new foods, and have a bad reaction, how do you know which food(s) is/are the culprit(s)? Is it 1 new food? Or 2? Or more? Or is it a toxic combination created by the mixing of several new foods? Do you drop the new diet immediately, or suffer along with it, hoping that things will improve? What are the risks? Why are you putting yourself through this? Do you think you can stick to an awful diet, lose weight, then go back to your old eating habits and *not* gain the weight back? Perhaps there is a better way. CUSTOMIZE YOURSELF is a better way.

## Getting Started And Staying In The Game

Diving head-first into a different or unusual new set of habits is not only challenging, stressful and possibly dangerous, but it makes bailing out altogether more attractive. Think about everyone you know who has begun a new diet. How many stick to it? How many decide they want to go back to eating what they loved before the new diet banned them from enjoying it? Every gym I have ever spent time in gets packed with new members in January, then thins out in February. With the best intentions, many people make a New Year's resolution to go the gym, but quit when their misery index exceeds their better judgement. The CUSTOMIZE YOURSELF approach provides antidotes to rushing in and out of potentially worthy, new health and fitness endeavors.

## Running From The Womb

When did you learn how to run? Did you bolt out of your mother's womb, sprint out of the hospital, and run a marathon? Probably not. It took a while to become a runner. Some rolling around, a helpful hand, some wobbly steps, then a progression from walking to running. It was a challenging journey that took time and effort, but you made it! Some bumps and bruises along the way, but the payoff was huge!

21

It's also a very early lesson in how to CUSTOMIZE YOURSELF. A journey of a thousand miles begins with a single step. So said Lao-tzu, or as many scholars have interpreted his text, *The journey of a thousand miles starts beneath your feet.* You have to first get up on your feet even before you can begin your journey.

## Who's Your Philosopher?

Gather the proverbs and phrases of those who inspire you, and may support, guide, smooth, invigorate, transform or redirect your journey. Philosophers, songwriters, poets, artists and achievers of all sorts are good sources. If I ever go into the T-shirt trade, or wallpaper business, I've got plenty to plaster. If you need a hook to hang your hat and scarf on, Voltaire, Campbell and West (not a law firm) offer their devices,

*I don't believe people are looking for the meaning of life as much as they are looking for the experience of being alive.*
*-Joseph Campbell*

*God gave us the gift of life; it is up to us to give ourselves the gift of living well.*
*-Voltaire*

*You only live once, but if you do it right, once is enough.*

*-Mae West*

The concept of a life well-lived is vast. Voltaire lived in Paris (1694-1778). New Yorkers Joseph Campbell (1904-1987) and Mae West (1893-1980) were born later, and traveled in different circles, but in close proximity. Mae was attracted to younger men. Perhaps they shared a dance, or a glance, across a crowded room?

The words of wise men and women can guide us, or derail us.

*What's past is prologue.*
*-William Shakespeare*

Or is it? Do you follow a script, or do you write your own? Do you run with the pack, or go solo? The choice is yours, and you can enrich your journey if you do some cherry-picking from the masters along the way.

Inspiration, insight and revelation may also be discovered, stumbled upon, or tripped over backwards in surprising, unusual or unlikely places. I thought Maryville, Missouri native Dale Carnegie was strictly for squares, until I read his work. His HOW TO WIN FRIENDS AND INFLUENCE PEOPLE[11] is a practical guide for creating good vibes while advancing human and business relations. His positive outlook and sound advice is as useful today as when published in 1936. You don't have to be a corporate animal to benefit from it.

---

[11]Dale Carnegie, *How to Win Friends and Influence People.* New York: Simon and Schuster, 1936.

Going back a little further, and about 7,000 miles over to the other side of the planet, for insight and inspiration, flip through Lao-tzu's TAO TE CHING. Written around the time of Confucius (551-479 B.C.E.), Lao-tzu's wisdom and counsel endure. Understanding consequences, achieving self-reliance, and the logic of good deeds are illuminated with simplicity and elegance.

If you take your journey one step at a time, you can pause and soak up your surroundings, adjust your direction, and confidently move forward. You can easily fine-tune, enjoy and perpetuate your new, customized self.

## The Order Of Things

This book is part of an ongoing series that aims to develop your own CUSTOMIZE YOURSELF program to integrate nutrition, fitness, mindbody connection, and longevity. There's plenty of overlap in these areas, but I put them in this order because my first impression was that if you engage the CUSTOMIZE YOURSELF approach to nutrition, it's easy to apply the same logic to fitness, mindbody connection and longevity. These are inextricably linked, and you may feel free to change 'The Order Of Things' as you please.

# Evolution

*Start by doing what's necessary, then do what's possible, and suddenly you are doing the impossible.*
*-St. Francis of Assisi*

CUSTOMIZE YOURSELF is designed to give you the tools to create and maintain a leaner, healthier, happier, less stressful, more vital and longer life. It doesn't demand that you weigh every morsel of food, time every workout, or record every step you take, although you're welcome to do it. It doesn't require that you become an Olympic athlete with 8% body fat, but if that's your goal, it shows how you can achieve it. Rather than set one or all of your goals at rapid-fire, 100% improvement, it will show you how to easily achieve a 25% improvement, and sustain it, instead of pouncing on a more lofty goal which you may boomerang from, while still retaining the option of going for a greater percentage in the future.

Think of yourself as a work in progress. No one is perfect. Desirable changes boost confidence, performance and self-esteem, enhance mindbody function, and can increase longevity. When I think about my flaws, my head spins, so I am quite grateful to be a work in progress. It gives me hope for the future. My own expedition to find health, fitness, happiness and longevity is a thread in this book, but it is not intended as an example for everyone to follow. You are welcome to draw from it, but I'm sure you will find more than a few things that I practice which are not perfectly suited to your itinerary.

The main purpose of this book is to inspire and guide you to customize your own journey, not to copy someone else's.

A lot of what I have learned is drawn from less-than-earth-shattering events from my life that have set me on a better course. As you read about them, think about your own experiences. Whatever you have encountered that has changed your behavior in any positive way is worth revisiting and exploring to help chart the path to create the new, customized you. Your personal history, both the good and the bad, is part of the process. Your life is unique and valuable. Learn from it and draw from it whatever supports your evolution.

So as we roll along, instead of glomming onto someone else's diet which you'll probably grow to hate and abandon, let's start with what you're eating now, and discover ways to evolve it into a better system, one that you can benefit from, love and embrace.

# Part I: *Plants And Animals*

# What Does Your Doctor Say?

Have you ever gone to a doctor, described a problem that you were having, and then the doctor asked you, "What do you eat?" If you live in the United States, the answer is, probably, never. I cannot think of a single time any medical doctor has ever asked me, "What do you eat?" In many parts of China, Hong Kong or Japan, that's the first question a doctor asks.

We are killing ourselves with the American diet. Heart disease in the United States has been the #1 killer for many decades. During the 1930s and 1940s, Western-trained doctors working at a large network of hospitals in sub-Saharan Africa discovered that heart disease practically did not exist in that region. Comparing autopsies of 632 individuals in Saint Louis, Missouri with 632 age-matched Ugandans, researchers found 136 Missourian deaths by heart attack, but zero heart attacks among the Ugandans.[12]

Many studies since have revealed that very low rates of heart disease still exist all over the world where plant-based diets predominate. By consuming greater amounts of grains, vegetables and fiber, and very little animal fat, rural populations in China and

---

[12] Michael Greger and Gene Stone, *How Not to Die*. New York: Flatiron Books, 2017, pp. 18-19.

Africa have shown total cholesterol levels averaging under 150 mg/dL.[13]

Many American doctors and health experts state that 200 mg/dL total cholesterol is a safe level. But is that the best plan while heart disease remains the leading cause of death for men and women in the United States? In 2020, it was estimated that one person died every 37 seconds from cardiovascular disease, translating into about 647,000 deaths for the year, or 1 in every 4 deaths.[14] The cost of heart disease health care services, medicines and productivity losses in the United States is estimated to be more than $219 billion.[15] And those costs and deaths will continue to rise unless American eating habits improve. Why not turn to more plant-based alternatives, and aim for total cholesterol of 150 mg/dL, instead of 200 mg/dL?

---

[13] Ibid.

[14] "Heart Disease Facts," Centers for Disease Control and Prevention, last reviewed: Sept. 8, 2020. https://www.cdc.gov/heartdisease/facts.htm

[15] Ibid.

# Time Bomb In A Bun

"Time bomb in a bun," is what Dr. Todd Anderson of the University of Calgary, and director of the Libin Cardiovascular Institute of Alberta declared after testing the effects of fast food breakfast sandwiches on a group of healthy university students. The subjects consumed a pair of breakfast sandwiches containing 900 calories and 50 grams of fat. Then 2 hours later, their blood vessels' velocity time integral (VTI), or "how much blood flow you can get in your arm," was measured, and revealed that their VTI decreased by 15-20%. Anderson concluded that a one-day drop in VTI won't kill you, but regular consumption will cause fat to build up in the walls of your arteries which can cause atherosclerosis, a narrowing of the arteries linked to heart disease and stroke.[16]

Or, to put it another way, fast food may be a fast recipe for early death.

---

[16] QMI Agency, "Study dubs breakfast sandwich a 'time bomb in a bun,'" TORONTO SUN, Oct. 31, 2012. https://torontosun.com/2012/10/31/study-dubs-breakfast-sandwich-a-time-bomb-in-a-bun/wcm/2cab1f47-ba72-4cd7-9f98-1546bba536e1

According to numerous American[17] and Canadian[18] studies, diets including fast food/high-fat meals can also increase the risks of insulin resistance, show increased fat in the liver, cause oxidative stress and inflammation, and cardiovascular reactivity to stress which can lead to hypertension.[19]

And if you're still not convinced of the perils of fast food, then you should watch Morgan Spurlock's entertaining and informative, Oscar-nominated documentary, SUPER SIZE ME. For 30 days, Spurlock consumed nothing but items on the McDonald's menu. As his camera crew and a team of doctors observe his physical and mental deterioration, Spurlock risks death to make his point.

Whatever your consumption of fast food is today, you should reduce it. To head off cardiovascular disease, avoid fast food altogether. Give your arteries a break now. They'll thank you for it later.

---

[17] Michael Greger with Gene Stone, *How Not to Die*. New York: Flatiron Books, 2017, p. 25.

[18] QMI Agency, "Study dubs breakfast sandwich a 'time bomb in a bun,'" TORONTO SUN, Oct. 31, 2012. https://torontosun.com/2012/10/31/study-dubs-breakfast-sandwich-a-time-bomb-in-a-bun/wcm/2cab1f47-ba72-4cd7-9f98-1546bba536e1

[19] Deanna Minich, Ph.D., "The Power of One Meal to Make or Break Your Health," HUFFPOST, Aug. 16, 2017. https://www.huffpost.com/entry/the-power-of-one-meal-to-make-or-break-your-health_b_5994dcf4e4b056a2b0ef02f4

# Everything Is Bad For You

If you don't agree that 'Everything is Bad for You,' pick any 10 of the last decade's 50 bestselling books on nutrition, and make a list of all the foods that these books tell you not to eat. You'll likely find just about everything you eat is bad for you for one reason or another.

Perhaps blueberries and walnuts and a few other newly crowned "superfoods" will not be on the list. Many experts extol the benefits of eating blueberries and walnuts, and for most people, they are absolutely correct. But in my case, they are at the top of my, "Bad for Me" list because blueberries give me diarrhea, and walnuts make me vomit. And if they don't cause the same reactions in you, consider that non-organic blueberries are typically coated with pesticides. And don't forget that it takes about 5 gallons of water to produce 1 walnut. Ninety-nine percent of all US walnuts are grown in California where severe drought will likely cause practical and ethical problems with sustaining walnut production.[20] Most people who eat blueberries and walnuts will benefit from them for sure, but not everyone. I bring up these personal examples because if you pay attention to the reactions

---

[20] Alex Park, Julia Lurie, "It Takes How Much Water to Grow an Almond?!" MOTHER JONES, Feb. 24, 2014. https://www.motherjones.com/environment/2014/02/wheres-californias-water-going/

you have to all sorts of foods, you will discover your own, "Bad for Me" list. Use it to improve your diet, and look for alternative foods to replace the offenders on your list.

# What Likes You?

And what doesn't like you?

The more specifically and accurately you can answer these questions about yourself, the more you will benefit. These questions are more important to your health and happiness than, "What do you like?" You already know what you like. Some of it is good for you. Some of it is bad. It's up to you to be aware of which foods you are eating that are causing you more harm than good, and then modifying/improving your diet accordingly. Paying attention to what you eat, and how you feel after eating it is a simple habit that will pay a lifetime of dividends. It's is not quite enough to let your gut be your only guide, but your gut can tell you a lot.

Sometimes the answers are obvious, like with me and blueberries and walnuts. But sometimes the answers are not so apparent. I know this may sound ridiculous, but it took me 20 years to figure out that the acid and sugar blast from a glass of orange juice was wreaking havoc in my gut, every day! For as long I can remember, there was a glass of orange juice on the kitchen table every morning. Everyone in my family drank their orange juice every morning. Get your vitamin C. It's good for you! Right? I thought so. Every morning I drank my orange juice, and every morning I had a stomachache. I didn't think about it too much. It just seemed like that's what happens in the morning. You get a stomachache, then later on, it goes away. As a teenager, I chalked it up to the stress of going to school every day. Damn school! Wake up way too early, run around the house getting ready, race out the door, hotfoot it to school, and plop into your assigned seat seconds before the late bell rings, or you get detention. An Orwellian nightmare! I couldn't wait till I got out of school so my life could be better. But then again, I still got the stomachaches in the summer too. Why was that?

I remember trying out for the Columbia High School swim team in the school's ancient indoor pool (circa 1908). Recognized as the oldest indoor high school pool in New Jersey (if not North America), we were told that the water in that pool had never been changed, and it was rumored that the 1918 Spanish flu was still living in there. Somehow I also got a message not to eat before the first morning of tryouts. It was a stressful situation. And I always ate breakfast before going to school. Always. Leaving the house before eating breakfast? Who does such a thing? Maybe just a glass of orange juice, that couldn't hurt, could it? How about playing it really safe, maybe just half a glass? So I drank just half a glass of orange juice, no food, and I'm off to the tryout. And wow, was it stressful, and hard, and a killer, and one by one, you could see every kid at the tryout who had breakfast, barf on the side of the pool (at least they didn't barf into the pool). But not me, I only had a half a glass of orange juice. And then, after the last kid who barfed up his breakfast on the side of the pool finished barfing, I proceeded to barf up my half a glass of orange juice right along side of the other barfers.

But it still didn't occur to me that maybe I should stop drinking orange juice until I reached the advanced age of 20 years old, when one fine day, out the blue, I thought, hey, maybe having a stomachache every morning is not normal. Maybe I could do something about it. What if I didn't have a glass of orange juice one morning? So I tried it. No orange juice, followed by no stomachache! Wow! Why didn't I think of that sooner? I had no clue about the acid balance in my stomach, but it turns out that dumping a load of sugar and citric acid in there jacked it up to painful levels. I also got the first inkling that fruit juice, which is basically fruit with the pulp removed, caused problems. When you eat whole fruit, the pulp slows the absorption of the sugar. But the sugar in fruit juice has no pulp to slow its absorption, so the sugar jolt from a glass of OJ is similar to the jolt you get from a can of soda. Twelve ounces of orange juice has 12 teaspoons of sugar, approximately the same amount in 12 ounce can of Coke, or about 36 grams of carbs, which is considered around half of what you should consume in a day.[21] Add that to the citric acid in orange juice, and my stomach objected, painfully.

We'll get into all the problems caused by sugar, and the food companies who overload it into practically everything, but for now, let's just consider that eliminating fruit juices can make you healthier and feel a lot better. Whole fruit is the way to go. I eat an orange every day, and get even more nutritional benefits without the stomach pain. It took me a while longer to figure out that I shouldn't torture my gut with apple juice either. No more apple juice of any kind, just

---

[21] David Perlmutter, MD, "The #1 Reason to Avoid Orange Juice," davidperlmutter MD, May 24, 2014. https://www.drperlmutter.com/avoid-orange-juice/

firm, crunchy apples. The same goes for every fruit you consume, eat the whole fruit and not its juice!

# Is There A Diet You Can Stick To?

If you're convinced that there is a great diet that will make you leaner, happier, healthier, and extend your life, you should go for it. Just make sure that you will stick to it for the rest of your life, or the benefits will go away with the diet.

But how do you know that your new diet is really that good or safe or sustainable?

For almost a decade, U.S. NEWS & WORLD REPORT has published its annual 'Best Diets' report. Reviewed by a panel of 24 distinguished doctors, scientists and health experts, these reports scrutinize and evaluate all sorts of diets, and provide a valuable resource for anyone looking for diet information and recommendations.[22]

Their 2021 version ranked 39 diets. For the 4th consecutive year, their #1 Best Overall Diet was the Mediterranean Diet.[23] With low intake of red meat, sugar and saturated fat, and an emphasis on a

---

[22] U.S. News Staff, "U.S. News Reveals Best Diet Rankings for 2021," U.S. NEWS & WORLD REPORT, Jan. 4, 2021.
https://www.usnews.com/info/blogs/press-room/articles/2021-01-04/us-news-reveals-best-diet-rankings-for-2021

[23] "Best Diets Overall," U.S. NEWS & WORLD REPORT, 2021.
https://health.usnews.com/best-diet/best-diets-overall

variety of produce, nuts and seeds, you can throw in a glass of red wine to wash it down, and you have a good mix. No matter what your eating habits may be, it's worth familiarizing yourself with the Mediterranean Diet. It deserves its #1 ranking.

Some of the currently most popular diets did not fare so well in the 'Best Diets' rankings. The Paleo Diet, (the caveman diet), landed at #31, and the Keto Diet, which encourages weight loss via fat-burning, came in at #37, tied for next-to-last. While you can find numerous rabid fans of the Keto Diet, many experts have a low opinion of it. Dr. David Katz, founding director of the Yale University Prevention Research Center, finds it unhealthy and unsustainable, "Losing weight fast by using a severely restricted, silly, unbalanced diet inevitably leads to even faster weight regain."[24]   And Stanford professor Christopher Gardner, who does research on low-carb diets at Stanford Prevention Research Center said, "Most health professionals are concerned that the degree of carb restriction requires someone to cut out many of the foods that have been consistently recommended as being healthy: fruits, beans/legumes and whole intact grains."[25]

Before you even consider going a specific diet, listen to the arguments made by the defenders of different diets against each other, like say, the Vegan Diet vs. the Paleo Diet. It may be something like,

---

[24] Sandee LaMotte, "Experts say the keto isn't sustainable, so why is it so popular?" CNN, Jan. 5, 2020.
https://www.cnn.com/2020/01/05/health/keto-diet-day-wellness/index.html

[25] Ibid.

'we are convinced that the Paleo Diet will shorten your life and kill you.' Then, listen to the arguments made by defenders of the Paleo Diet against the Vegan Diet. Are they similar, if not identical?

For most people, abandoning their eating habits, and adopting a new diet is an unnerving proposition that they will not stick to. The British company Alpro, which advocates plant-based eating, did a survey of over 2,000 Brits and their dieting habits. About half of this group were regular dieters. Alpro found that 40% of dieters quit within the first 7 days, 20% lasted a month, 20% hung in for 3 months, and the rest stuck to it for at least 6 months. Only 5% were likely still be on their chosen diet after one year.[26] Are you a 5%-er?

UCLA researchers conducted a comprehensive analysis of 31 long-term diet studies, and concluded that dieting does not work. They found that most dieters would be better off not going on a diet at all. Most dieters regain all the weight they lost, plus more, and suffer wear and tear on their bodies in the process. Several of the studies they analyzed indicated that dieting is actually a consistent predictor of future weight gain. They also found evidence that repeatedly losing and gaining weight is linked to heart disease, stroke, diabetes and altered immune function.[27] Lead author of the UCLA study, Dr. Traci Mann, who now directs the University of Minnesota

---

[26] "Diet starts today... and ends on Friday: How we quickly slip back into bad eating habits within a few days," DAILY MAIL, Sept. 16, 2013. https://www.dailymail.co.uk/news/article-2421737/Diet-starts-today--ends-Friday-How-quickly-slip-bad-eating-habits-days.html

[27] Stuart Wolpert, "Dieting does not work, UCLA researchers report," UCLA NEWSROOM, Apr. 3, 2007. https://newsroom.ucla.edu/releases/Dieting-Does-Not-Work-UCLA-Researchers-7832

Health and Eating Laboratory,[28] has spent a career studying diets. In her book, SECRETS FROM THE EATING LAB, she points out that our bodies and brains are not hardwired to resist food. It goes against our biological imperative to survive. Relying on the notion of willpower to lose weight is an illusion. She advocates for moderation (like Mom), avoiding the dieting industry's mass marketing mayhem, smarter labeling, portion control, and socializing with people with healthy habits.[29]

Also bear in mind, drastic changes in diet can result in headaches, mood swings, physical or mental fatigue, digestive problems and other maladies.[30]

CUSTOMIZE YOURSELF advocates taking a good, honest look at your present diet, and improving it, in stages, one step at a time, like a journey of a thousand miles, beginning with the first step.

---

[28] The Mann Lab, University of Minnesota.
http://mannlab.psych.umn.edu/index.html

[29] Traci Mann, *Secrets from the Eating Lab,* New York: Harper Wave, 2015.

[30] Cynthia Sass, "5 Reasons Most Diets Fail Within 7 Days," HEALTH, Sept. 19, 2013. https://www.health.com/nutrition/5-reasons-most-diets-fail-within-7-days

## More Harm Than Good

Make a list of foods you typically eat which are likely to do you 'More Harm Than Good.' Include anything with added or excessive sugar, salt, fat, flour, chemicals, additives, preservatives, fried foods, desserts, highly-processed foods, and the like. If you're not sure about a particular item, put it to the list anyway. You can always remove it later. Next to each entry, put the number of times per week on average that you consume that food, e.g. BACON (3), DONUTS (2), ICE CREAM (1), FRENCH FRIES (4), and so on.

As you read this book, you can add or subtract items. It doesn't have to be a perfect list. You don't have weigh or measure anything. For now, leave 'Date' and 'Goal' blank. We'll come back to them later.

### MORE HARM THAN GOOD:

Food:_____ Date:_____ Goal:_____

Food:_____ Date:_____ Goal:_____

Food:_____ Date:_____ Goal:_____

Food:_____ Date:_____ Goal:_____

Food:_____ Date:_____ Goal:_____

Food:_____ Date:_____ Goal:_____

Food:_____ Date:_____ Goal:_____

Food:_____ Date:_____ Goal:_____

Food:_____ Date:_____ Goal:_____

Food:_____ Date:_____ Goal:_____

# French Fries And Married Guys

A simple way to talk yourself out of a mound of french fries is to ask yourself, would you feed them to your dog? No? Then why would you eat them?

If the only excuse you can come up is that you don't have a dog, I have an innocent tale of epiphany.

Way back in my sun-worshipping (and sun-burning) years, when I was a lifeguard on Point Pleasant Beach, New Jersey, all sorts of people would come up to the lifeguard stand and ask a great variety of questions. Some of it was obvious stuff like, is it safe to go swimming? Have you seen any sharks today? And some of them wanted to know more. I witnessed some serious adults ask clueless teenage lifeguards about what they should do with their lives. They got mostly unsatisfying answers. They would mumble some, "Yeah, sure, thanks," and trudge away. Then the lifeguard would turn to me and ask, "What the hell was I supposed to say, 'Leave your wife, quit your job, and get a surfboard?'" I wasn't much help, but we all realized that a few encouraging proverbs could benefit our lifesaving lexicon.

Without crediting Lao-tzu, we tried, "A journey of a thousand miles begins with a single step." And then, "A bird in the hand is worth two in the bush." Another was, "A chain is only as strong as its weakest link." To avoid disaster, "Don't cross that bridge until you come to it." It was obvious that we were not saving humanity. I mean, that's what lifeguards do. We save lives. Or at least we save people from drowning. Saving souls, or providing wise counsel was surely beyond our pay grade. But since we were mostly sitting on our asses for 8 hours a day, we had the time and space to delve deeper. A new, popular-on-the-beach proverb became, "We'll burn that bridge when we come to it." Then, "The early bird catches the worm, but who likes worms?" After that, "If ain't broke, break it." We tried, "Where there's a will, there's relatives." And then there was, "It's no use crying over spilt milk, but beer is different, you can cry over spilt beer." One of the beach managers had a solution for every problem, "Let's play it by ear." I'm still trying to figure out that one.

Most of our proverb-ial-efforts were pretty lame, but we eventually came up with one that stuck. Lifeguards, for some strange reason, often attract very young girls, too young to be accurate, who gather at the stand, perched at the feet of wind-swept, teenage gods who protect the community from the angry sea. And these way too-young girls act terribly interested, and ask a bunch of their own strange questions, and way, way before they turn 18, disappear over the western horizon because they eventually realize that they couldn't care less about a bunch of barely-sentient, sit-for-a-living-to-get-a-paid-tan, minor league hedonists who were totally broke all the time because they squandered their petty wages on cheap beer and bad pot. Anyway, before all that went down, we flawed lifeguards felt a shred of adult responsibility to give some brotherly advice to our  young sisters. And the line that stuck was,

*Stay away from french fries and married guys.*
*-Anon. lifeguard, circa 1970-something*

Nothing profound mind you, but it stuck, and summer after summer, it was best advice we had to give. I bring it up now because french fries and fried foods in general are really bad for everybody. The connections between eating fried foods and obesity and heart disease have become well established. A 2017 study by Dr. Nicola Veronese at the Institute of Clinical Research and Education in Medicine in Padova, Italy, concluded that, among 4,440 people, ages 45 to 79, those who ate french fries, fried potatoes and hash browns more than twice a week were more likely to die early than those who ate them less often.[31] We may gather that the eminent doctor would probably agree with the findings of some late 20th century professional chair-sitters who warned young maidens about the perils of french fries (and married guys).

Now, let's go back to your 'MORE HARM THAN GOOD' list. How many times a week do you eat fried foods? Two? Five? Ten? Whatever it is, right now, this minute, make a pledge to reduce this number. Let's say you eat french fries 4 times a week. OK, your pledge is to cut down to 3 times a week. That's it. Just once a week, you'll refrain from french fries. It's easy. You can do it. Even if there may come a non-french fries day upon which you're struck by

---

[31] Stephanie Watson, "How Bad for Your Are Fried Foods?" WebMD, June 17, 2017. https://www.webmd.com/diet/news/20170622/how-bad-for-you-are-fried-foods

a terrible jones for french fries, relax, you can have them the next day. And you will have them. And they will taste even better. I promise.

If you swore right now to never eat a french fry again, that would be fantastic! You think you can do that? If you can do it, you would be so special. And rare. What discipline. I am so impressed. You just added years to your life. And more vitality. And wow, you look better too!

But let's face it, you love french fries. You're weak. You don't have amazing, mind-blowing discipline. Right? Setting an unrealistic goal for yourself is setting yourself up for failure. You don't want that. So what do you do? You set a realistic goal, an easily achievable and sustainable goal. By skipping the fries just once a week, you have just reduced your french fry intake by 25%. Twenty-five percent of all that french fry grease and sludge will not enter your body. That is fantastic! If you do not adopt or follow a single suggestion from the rest of this book, you will have accomplished an important and significant achievement in making yourself a healthier person. Congratulations!

On your 'MORE HARM THAN GOOD LIST,' next to "FRENCH FRIES," write down today's date, and your goal, "25% LESS."

Now, you only have one more thing to do. It'll only take a few seconds. Mark on your calendar, 6 months from today, "25% LESS FRIES" That is your 6 month anniversary. When you arrive at this special date, you will celebrate! Visualize the massive pile of 26 fried food sludge portions that you did not torture your body with, that you are not lugging around on your gut hanging over your pants, and celebrate! Throw a party for the new, customized you. You have eliminated a weekly load of grease, and done it for 6 months straight!

Then, mark on your on your calendar, 6 months further down the road, "25% LESS FRIES", and throw yourself another party, a one-whole-year anniversary party. Good for you, you've earned it!

Or, if you like… and this is totally optional… you really don't have to do it… but you may want to consider… just consider… don't act… just think about the idea of perhaps reducing your fried sludge intake by another 25%. You don't have to do it. You may not want to do it. If you don't want to do it, by all means, don't do it. But just consider it. Since you knocked off 25% 6 months ago, you know you have the ability to ban another fraction of that mountain of grease weighing you down. If you're happy with original 25% reduction, and enjoyed the party you threw for yourself, (and by the way, you can have a fried-grease-reduction bash every 6 months for the rest of your life), do nothing. But if the idea of having a party in 6 months to celebrate a *50%* reduction in ugly sludge appeals to you, WOW, you can have even a bigger and better party! And, you will be thrilled to mark, "50% LESS FRIES."

Whether or not you go for the 50% milestone, you have clearly demonstrated and proved to yourself how easy it is to successfully apply and sustain the 25%-at-a-time, slow-and-steady-wins-the-game, I-can-do-this-for-the-rest-of-my-life, CUSTOMIZE YOURSELF system to your own well-being.

And if you so desire, this simple process can be applied to every item on your 'MORE HARM THAN GOOD' list that you know or learn about, or decide for any reason, is not good for you. It works for donuts, chips, bacon and every other unhealthy entry on your list.

If you have ever bailed out of a diet, or have any doubts about your ability to make positive changes and stick to them, don't attack all items on your 'MORE HARM THAN GOOD' list all at once. Take your time. Do it methodically. If you feel you need to build your confidence slowly, you can wait for weeks or even months between making the 25% cut on item #1, and then applying it to the next offender on your list. Again, if you only make that one 25% reduction of your fried food intake, and do nothing else, you have reached a significant milestone, and made a lasting and valuable improvement!

## My Own Fried Food Saga

Nowadays, on average, I eat fried food about once or twice a year. Usually, it's because I find myself in a how-did-I-get-stuck-in-this-place restaurant with an archaic, unenlightened menu that's so disappointing and frustrating, the best compromised order I can come up with still has grease.

While I may have consumed about a billion french fries as a voracious child, I can safely say that I would be very happy to never eat a french fry again. And to validate the CUSTOMIZE YOURSELF process, it's only fair that I relate how I got the french fry monkey off my back. Truth be told, when I was a kid, I tried to eat french fries every day. Man, did I crave fries! In a good week, I might figure out how to get my greasy little hands on those fries 5 or 6 times. I would pile them on a hamburger, dip them in ice cream, or just drown 'em in ketchup. If I was in a restaurant that had fried onion rings, I'd get them too. If I was low on cash (most of the time), I'd have a trusty friend split an order. French fries *and* fried onion rings, man oh man, serious grease! On Fridays, my mother would make fried chicken, (putting the "Fri" in Fridays). On Saturday, we'd have leftover chicken, more grease! And for in-between-grease, I could always make an emotional plea (i.e. annoying whine) for potato chips, corn chips, cheese doodles or anything in a bag that looked like it might have grease in it.

Life was good. I was filled with grease, and my taste buds were screaming for more. And then, I started noticing something. It was shortly after I realized that orange juice sugar and citric acid were roiling my gut. I quit the OJ, and lost the morning stomachache, but it became apparent that later in the day, I didn't feel all that great after eating a mound of fries. It wasn't like the pain of the OJ, it was just that I felt much better when I skipped the fries. And the fried onion rings were even worse. They churned more than the french fries. What a cruel world! Did I damage my gut with too much grease? Did a lifetime of orange juice foul up my grease processor? Or maybe I was just lucky that I was beginning to learn how to monitor myself, and make healthy adjustments.

I learned a little more about fried foods, and even back then, it wasn't hard to figure out how fattening and unhealthful they were. So I cut down on the fries. I cut out the onion rings. I reduced my chip consumption. And I felt better. I realized that I like baked potatoes as much as fried potatoes, so not long after, I quit the french fries altogether. For quite some time afterwards, I still bought a large bag of chips on each visit to the supermarket. Eventually I noticed that I didn't feel so wonderful after eating the chips either. And while the chips were tasty, I was never satisfied. I could eat a few or a ton, and still,

*I can't get no satisfaction*
*I can't get no satisfaction*
*Cause I try and I try and I try and I try*

*I can't get no, I can't get no*[32]


    The Stones got me off the chips. The next time I went to the market, cruising the massive chip aisle, Dionne Warwick sang to me,


*Walk on by (don't stop)…*
*Walk on by (don't stop)…*[33]


    I just pushed my cart right past the chips… and kept going. I never turned back. I didn't buy chips that week, or the following week, or ever. It's been decades of not buying chips. I don't miss them. I don't want them. I don't need them. They're not good for me. And now, I don't even like them![34]

---

[32]The Rolling Stones. "(I Can't Get No) Satisfaction." RCA Records, 1965.

[33] Dionne Warwick. "Walk On By." *Make Way for Dionne Warwick.* Scepter. 1964. Coincidentally, Dionne Warwick lived in Maplewood, New Jersey at this time.

[34] Thanks to Mick Jagger, Keith Richards, Dionne Warwick, Burt Bachrach and Hal David.

# The Meat Section

I had a craving for meat in my youth that was even more powerful than my french fry addiction. I had to have meat twice a day or my head would explode. Meat for lunch and dinner was required, breakfast was optional. If I had to settle for a hamburger or hot dog, I would become distracted, and count the minutes before the next sizzling steak or rare roast beef would be up for grabs. I would jones constantly for all sorts of deli meats. Corned beef with just the right amount of fat was the ultimate, but white meat turkey sliced so thin that it was translucent when held up to the sun, or pastrami sliced just a little thicker, or paper thin cold roast beef, filled and crowded my fantasies. And don't forget the swiss cheese, mandatory on the roast beef, optional on the turkey, forbidden on corned beef. These were the obsessions of a pre-orgasmic kid who had no clue that these food desires would soon have to compete for attention with the onset of puberty. They didn't go away of course, just made life more challenging.

As I was doing my best to promulgate spectacular deli meat consumption, I barely noticed that, while there was an extensive array of Jewish delicatessens all over New Jersey and New York,[35] they

---

[35] Early 20th century statistics are spotty, but in 1931, there were 1,550 Kosher delis in New York City alone.

were pretty much nonexistent, basically unknown in other parts of the country. I remember when my brother, Marc was an officer in the U.S Public Health Service, assigned to a post on the Zuni reservation in New Mexico, the only complaint we ever heard way back east was that the nearest corned beef was in Phoenix, Arizona, at a distance of 293 miles, which could be reached in 5 hours, but only if you crushed the gas pedal and made no stops. And he made no stops.

Nowadays, outside of Brooklyn, it's pretty hard to find a Kosher deli.[36] Their demise is connected to a variety of factors regarding changing tastes and nutritional awareness, but I have my own meshuga theory. The proliferation of Jewish delis in the suburban expansions of the 1950s, 60s and 70s created such wealth among the owners of these establishments that they sent their kids to expensive medical schools where many of them became cardiologists to serve the growing needs of their parents' customers. And that feedback loop eventually resulted in the diminution of the Jewish deli industry. In the ensuing battles between the cardiologists and the corned beef, the cardiologists gained the upper hand, and the corned beef lost out. The cardiologists' patients ate less corned beef, and the cardiologists' parents sold less corned beef. I suppose if we really needed to know more about the rise and fall of corned beef in America, there might be

---

Leo Schwartz, "Keeping it Kosher," ROADS & KINGDOMS, Oct. 9, 2019. https://roadsandkingdoms.com/2019/keeping-it-kosher/

[36] In 2018, it was estimated that there were only about 20 Jewish delis left in New York. Tzach Yoked, "The Rise and Fall of the Old New York Jewish Deli," HAARETZ, Jan. 16, 2018. https://www.haaretz.com/us-news/.premium.MAGAZINE-new-deli-the-rise-and-fall-and-rise-of-the-old-n-y-jewish-deli-1.5730860

a medical anthropologist willing to pursue further study. However, such a lark could be tempered by some sobering findings by the World Health Organization International Agency for Research on Cancer (IARC). On the subject of red meat, the IARC has stated, "After thoroughly reviewing the accumulated scientific literature, a Working Group of 22 experts from 10 countries convened by the IARC Monographs Programme classified the consumption of red meat as probably carcinogenic to humans. This association was observed mainly for colorectal cancer, but associations were also seen for pancreatic cancer and prostate cancer." Regarding processed meat (sorry corned beef, this includes you), the IARC stated, "Processed meat was classified as carcinogenic to humans (Group 1), based on sufficient evidence in humans that the consumption of processed meat causes colorectal cancer." They also concluded that each 50 gram portion (1.8 ounces) of processed meat eaten daily increases the risk of colorectal cancer by 18%.[37]

Even today, you can find delis in America that claim to pile on 12-16 ounces of corned beef on a single sandwich. Also note, one strip of bacon (average thickness) weighs about 1.1 ounces.[38] You do the math.

---

[37] IARC Monographs evaluate consumption of red meat and processed meat," International Agency Research on Cancer, World Health Organization, press release, Oct . 26, 2015.  https://www.iarc.fr/wp-content/uploads/2018/07/pr240_E.pdf

[38] Peggy Trowbridge Filippone, "Bacon Equivalents and Substitutions," THE SPRUCE EATS, Updated: Sept. 27, 2019..
https://www.thespruceeats.com/bacon-equivalents-and-substitutions-1807458

Back in the meat-crazed 1970s, I took what was touted as the first general course in Ecology at Washington University in St. Louis, Missouri, where I began to learn about some of the negative aspects of meat consumption. Americans' rising cholesterol levels were directly connected to the increasing ingestion of meat, milk, cheese, butter and other animal products, along with less active lifestyles; and it was communicated that the road to heart disease, the #1 killer in America, was paved with steak, roast beef, corned beef, hamburgers, hot dogs, ham and bacon, (the rap on dairy came later), with a clear implication that reducing meat consumption would slash one's chances of being iced by America's #1 killer.

It was also taught way back then that it took 8 pounds of grain to make 1 pound of beef, and if we dedicated just a portion of that grain to feeding people instead of cows, we could wipe out starvation in the world.

At that time, the world's population was 3.7 billion. Now, with population about to cross the 8 billion mark (unless altered by pandemics, climate disasters, wars, genocide and a variety of other murderous activity), the demand for meat has vastly increased, and so has the accompanying resource depletion. Besides those 8 pounds of grain, it takes about 2,500 gallons of water, 35 pounds of topsoil and 1 gallon of gasoline, to produce that 1 pound of beef. Seventy percent of US grain production is fed to livestock. Five million acres of rainforest are wiped out annually in South and Central America alone to create cattle pasture. America's farm animals produce 10 times more waste than humans, causing extensive water pollution.[39]

---

[39] "Food Choices and the Planet," EarthSave.
http://www.earthsave.org/environment.htm

Overgrazing is the most pervasive cause of desertification in the world.[40] And localized meat-caused pollution hotspots abound, e.g. more soot is emitted from the grills of Los Angeles fast food restaurants than all the city buses.[41]

Stanford University Global Carbon Project co-author Rob Jackson warns that global carbon dioxide ($CO_2$) levels in our atmosphere, "are now higher than they've been for millions of years."[42] While global transport (primarily road, rail, air and marine transportation) accounts for 24 percent of global $CO_2$ emissions,[43] $CO_2$ emissions from global livestock add up to 14.5 percent of all $CO_2$ emissions.[44]

Cows and pigs burping and farting are just not as funny as they used to be. But reducing tooting is not impossible. In 2016, the Union of Concerned Scientists scorecard of major beef sellers' deforestation

---

[40] Myra Klockenbrink, "The New Range War Has the Desert as Foe," *New York Times,* Aug. 20, 1991, p. 3.

[41] *San Jose Mercury News*, Sept. 6, 1994

[42] Doyle Rice, "Emissions of carbon dioxide into Earth's atmosphere reach record high," USA TODAY, Updated: Dec. 6, 2018. https://www.usatoday.com/story/news/world/2018/12/05/carbon-dioxide-earths-atmosphere-soars-highest-level-millions-years/2215508002/

[43] Shiying Wang, Mengpin Ge, "Everything You Need to Know About the Fastest-Growing Source of Global Emissions: Transport" WORLD RECOURCES INSTITUTE, Oct. 16, 2019. https://www.wri.org/blog/2019/10/everything-you-need-know-about-fastest-growing-source-global-emissions-transport

[44] "Key facts and findings, By the numbers: GHG emissions by livestock," Food and Agriculture Organization of the United Nations. http://www.fao.org/news/story/en/item/197623/icode/

practices gave Burger King a *zero*, putting them far behind other large offenders like Wal-Mart, McDonald's and Wendy's.[45] In 2020, after years of criticism from advocacy organizations, Burger King announced a program to add lemongrass to some of their cows' feed, claiming a 33% reduction in methane emissions from those lucky cows.[46] If this program is successful, and expanded, and adopted by many other companies, it could be meaningful. Concerned citizens and corporate investors should join environmental advocates to demand better practices by the big meat sellers.

If the experts on animal gas want a broader perspective, perhaps they can apply their research to analyze the effects of human farting too. It could be an entertaining dissertation topic. Might clear the air.

---

[45] "Flunking the Planet, America's Leading Food Companies Fail on Sustainable Meat" MIGHTY EARTH. https://www.mightyearth.org/wp-content/uploads/2018/08/Flunking-the-Planet-Americas-Leading-Food-Companies-Fail-on-Sustainable-Meat.pdf

[46] Jordan Valkinsky, "Burger King's latest sustainability effort: reduce cow farts," CNN BUSINESS, July 14, 2020. https://www.cnn.com/2020/07/14/business/burger-king-cow-diet/index.html

# The Factory Meat Section

It's fair to say that factory meat is toxic. You should avoid it. If you do eat meat, stick to grass-fed, and keep the portions small.

Almost all of the meat consumed in the United States is factory meat. While 75% of U.S. adults believe that they typically buy "humane products," only 1 percent of farmed animals are raised on non-factory farms.[47] Using data from the USDA Census of Agriculture, the Sentience Institute has estimated that 70.4% of cows, 98.3% of pigs, 99.8% of turkeys, 98.2% of chickens raised for eggs, and over 99.9% of chickens raised for meat are living in factory farms.[48]

These animals are typically fed grain that contains pesticides, along with hormones and antibiotics. Many are fed other animal parts (that could be their relatives). U.S. chickens are dipped in chlorinated water after slaughter to kill bacteria that has grown on them as a result

---

[47] Liam Gilliver, ""99% of US Farmed Animals Live On Factory Farms, Study Says," PLANT BASED NEWS, Updated: Sept. 28, 2020. https://www.plantbasednews.org/culture/factory-farms-study

[48] Jacy Reese Anthis, "US Factory Farming Estimates," SCIENCE INSTITUTE, Updated Apr. 11, 2019. https://www.sentienceinstitute.org/us-factory-farming-estimates

of the birds, "literally sitting in each other's waste."[49] Yum! (Until recently, arsenic was commonly fed to chickens).[50]

Factory meat production is a cruel, inhumane, hellish environment where a sick animal just can't raise a hoof or a claw, and request a visit to the vet. They just get mixed in with the rest. Crowding animals in gruesome conditions is practically a formula to instill viruses, and encourage them to spread, and become more virulent.

We are at risk of more pandemics not only because wild bats are being crowded out of their environments by humans destroying their habitats, and migration caused by climate change, and the dangers posed by wet markets in Asia. Factory farms also create conditions where a virus like COVID-19 or SARS can make the jump from animals to humans. According to Michael Greger, author of BIRD FLU: A VIRUS OF OUR OWN HATCHING, "If you actually want to create global pandemics, then build factory farms."[51]

As COVID-19 quickly spread across the United States, mistreatment of workers at meat plants exacerbated the horror. Many workers are immigrants, almost all are low-wage and poorly

---

[49] Sophie Kevany, "US chickens 'literally sitting in each other's waste' says RSPCA," THE GUARDIAN, Aug. 17, 2020.
https://www.theguardian.com/environment/2020/aug/17/us-chickens-literally-sitting-in-each-others-waste-says-rspca-brexit

[50] Wenonah Hauter, "Big Pharma Cover Up: Hiding Significant Levels of Arsenic in Your Chicken," ECOWATCH, Nov. 21, 2019.
https://www.ecowatch.com/big-pharma-cover-up-hiding-significant-levels-of-arsenic-in-your-chick-1881975113.html

[51] Michael Greger, *Bird Flu: A Virus of Our Hatching.* New York: Lantern Books, 2006.

educated. Repetitive-motion, 12-hour shifts are common.[52] [53] The United States Department of Labor Occupational Safety and Health Administration (OSHA) describes a long list of health and safety hazards plaguing the meat packing industry including, "exposure to high noise levels, dangerous equipment, slippery floors, musculoskeletal disorders, and hazardous chemicals (including ammonia that is used as a refrigerant). Musculoskeletal disorders comprise a large part of these serious injuries and continue to be common among meat packing workers. In addition, meat packing workers can be exposed to biological hazards associated with handling live animals or exposures to feces and blood which can increase their risk for many diseases."[54]

According to OSHA data covering only 22 of the 50 states, from 2015 to 2017 there were 550 serious injuries. Amputations happen on average twice a week.[55] When COVID-19 struck, thousands of

---

[52] Polly Mosendz, Peter Waldman, Lydia Mulvany, "U.S. Meat Plants Are Deadly as Ever, With No Incentive to Change," BLOOMBERG BUSINESSWEEK, June 18, 2020. https://www.bloomberg.com/news/features/2020-06-18/how-meat-plants-were-allowed-to-become-coronavirus-hot-spots?srnd=premium

[53] "Factory Farm Workers," FOOD EMPOWERMENT PROJECT. https://foodispower.org/human-labor-slavery/factory-farm-workers/

[54] "Meatpacking," United State Department of Labor, OSHA. https://www.osha.gov/SLTC/meatpacking/index.html

[55] Andrew Wasley, Christopher Cook, Natalie Jones, "Two amputations a week: the cost of working in a US meat plant," THE GUARDIAN, July 5, 2018. https://www.theguardian.com/environment/2018/jul/05/amputations-serious-injuries-us-meat-industry-plant

workers tested positive, forcing plant closings, and causing extensive human suffering and death.

Factory farms not only pose viral pandemic risks like those of COVID-19 and the 1918 influenza pandemic, but also bacterial pandemic risks like the Black Death (bubonic plague) that raged for hundreds of years. PANDEMIC[56] author Sonia Shah noted, "When I was writing my book, I asked my sources what keeps them awake at night. They usually had two answers: virulent avian influenza and highly drug-resistant forms of bacterial pathogens. Both those things are driven by the crowding in factory farms. These are ticking time bombs."[57]

The issue of antibiotic resistance is worsened by animal farmers using mass quantities of antibiotics on livestock and poultry. While the Centers for Disease Control and Prevention (CDC) has estimated that antibiotic-resistant infections cause 50,000 death a year, a University of Washington study says that this number could be as high as 162,000 deaths per year. Hospitals may be drastically underreporting these deaths because the infections were acquired in their facilities, which could make them look bad and hurt their business. (Causes of death could be listed as cancer or "underlying factors" to cover up). In 2018 and 2019, pharmaceutical companies like Achaogen, Aradigm, Tetraphase Pharmaceuticals and Melinta

---

[56]Sonia Shah, *Pandemic*. New York: Sarah Crichton Books, 2016.

[57] Sigal Samuel, 'The meat we eat is a pandemic risk, too," VOX, Updated Aug. 20, 2020. https://www.vox.com/future-perfect/2020/4/22/21228158/coronavirus-pandemic-risk-factory-farming-meat

Therapeutics received FDA approvals for new antibiotics only to see their businesses wiped out due to lack of government support. This is because new antibiotics are used only as a last resort, and must be used sparingly to tamp down the progression of antibiotic resistance, so they cannot be sold in large volumes, preventing drug companies from recovering their costs, and driving them out of business. Not only has our market-driven economy failed to invest in virus-preventing and fighting efforts, research and equipment (e.g. COVID-19), the same failure is happening in the lack-of-fight against bacterial and fungal infections. Without new therapies, the United Nations estimates that worldwide deaths could reach 10,000,000 by 2050.[58] [59] [60]

The elimination of factory farms should not be a partisan issue. Even before COVID-19 started spreading, Senator Cory Booker (D-NJ), and Representative Tulsi Gabbard (D-HI) introduced legislation placing a moratorium on large factory farms, phasing them out by 2040.[61] In response, the conservative NATIONAL REVIEW

---

[58] Paul Solman, "As a virus ravages the world, antibiotic makers are in disarray," PBS NEWS HOUR, July 29, 2020. Transcript: https://www.pbs.org/newshour/show/as-a-virus-ravages-the-world-antibiotic-makers-are-in-disarray

[59] "Why is so hard to develop new antibiotics?" Wellcome, Jan. 21, 2020. https://wellcome.ac.uk/news/why-is-it-so-hard-develop-new-antibiotics

[60] Andrew Jacobs, "Crisis Looms in Antibiotics as Drug Makers Go Bankrupt," THE NEW YORK TIMES, Dec. 25, 2019. https://www.nytimes.com/2019/12/25/health/antibiotics-new-resistance.html

[61] "Booker Unveils Bill to Reform Farm System," booker.senate.gov, Dec. 16, 2019. https://www.booker.senate.gov/news/press/booker-unveils-bill-to-reform-farm-system

supported Booker's Farm System Reform Bill, "Senator Booker Is Right about Factory Farming," noting that the H1N1 "swine flu" which killed over 12,000 Americans and hospitalized 274,000 likely originated in American factory farms, and the probability of more pandemics only increases as long as factory farms continue to exist.[62] [63] [64] The phase-out of factory farms can happen much faster if we stop eating factory meat.

And since you've already cut your french fries consumption down by 25%, it's just as easy to do the same thing with meat. If you eat meat 8 times a week, make it 6. If you eat meat 4 times a week, make it 3. On your 'MORE HARM THAN GOOD LIST,' next to "MEAT," write down today's date, and your goal, "25% LESS." Then, note on your calendar 6 months from now, "25% LESS MEAT." And, throw yourself another party. You'll deserve it.

And don't forget, and this is totally optional, you don't have to do it, but you may want to consider the idea of reducing your meat intake

---

[62] Spencer Case, "Senator Booker Is Right about Factory Farming," NATIONAL REVIEW, Apr. 6, 2020.
https://www.nationalreview.com/magazine/2020/04/06/senator-booker-is-right-about-factory-farming/

[63] Sigal Samuel, "The meat we eat is a pandemic risk, too," VOX, Updated Aug. 20, 2020. https://www.vox.com/future-perfect/2020/4/22/21228158/coronavirus-pandemic-risk-factory-farming-meat

[64] Dylan Matthews, "Factory farms abuse workers, animals, and the environment. Cory Booker has a plan to stop them." VOX, Dec. 20, 2019. https://www.vox.com/future-perfect/2019/12/20/21028200/factory-farms-abuse-workers-animals-and-the-environment-cory-booker-has-a-plan-to-stop-them

by another 25%. If you're happy with original 25% reduction, and enjoyed the 2 parties you threw for yourself, (and by the way, you can have a meat-reduction bash every 6 months for the rest of your life), do nothing. But if the idea of having a party in 6 months to celebrate a 50% reduction in meat intake appeals to you, WOW, you can have even a bigger and better "50% LESS MEAT" party!

Whether or not you go for the 50% milestone, you have clearly demonstrated and proved to yourself how to successfully apply and sustain the 25%-at-a-time, slow-and-steady-wins-the-game, I-can-do-this, CUSTOMIZE YOURSELF system to your own well-being once again. Congratulations!

To reduce cancer risk, pandemic threats, and the dangers of climate change, we must seriously address meat consumption. Bottom line, save your arteries, save your life, save the planet, eat less meat!

# Going Cold Turkey With Meat

My own escape from factory meat had a festive ending. In 1983, while I was unconsciously employing the CUSTOMIZE YOURSELF gradual reduction approach, and nearing ground zero, I got a cheap ticket to the Carnival in Rio de Janeiro. The excitement of attending the world's biggest party also provided an opportunity to sample a whole new menu in a distant locale. My plan was to eat seafood, coconuts and/or whatever-the-hell else the Brazilians ate besides meat.

Even with inflation raging at over 100%, (and I still can't imagine how they got through that), I quickly discovered that my extremely limited dollars would not go very far in Rio. With seafood and shrimp starting at 7 bucks a plate, I would burn through my cash too quickly. However, at practically any sidewalk café, you could buy a filet mignon for 3 U.S. dollars! And it was not just any filet mignon. It was the most tender, mouth-watering filet you could imagine. In fact, it was so tender, you could eat it with a spoon. There was nothing like this back in the meat-wild USA. So, for 9 days straight, I ate the some of the best meat in the Western Hemisphere. I had my fill. That's the last time I ate meat.

I don't miss meat at all. I have no desire to eat meat ever again. At this point, I doubt I even have adequate enzymes to digest it. It would be like eating a shoe. In fact, nowadays, a shoe is about as appetizing to me as a piece of meat. The food I craved and gorged on as a child is now simply a soon-to-be rotting slab of animal flesh that could just as easily be categorized as a by-product of a shoe.

You don't have to flee to Brazil to change your eating habits, but any creative enterprise that will help your achieve your goals and CUSTOMIZE YOURSELF is worth pursuing. Use your imagination. Plan an adventure which takes you into a new or different environment, and consider how you may enhance it by incorporating your new CUSTOMIZE YOURSELF tools.

# The Rap On Dairy

For decades, dairy industry lobbyists have colluded with government officials to find ways to use taxpayer dollars to promote dairy consumption. Beside making soda industry lobbyists jealous, they have managed to convince most Americans that they must consume significant amounts of dairy products in order to survive. As I write this, the U.S. Department of Agriculture states on their website, "The amount of dairy foods you need to eat depends on your age. The amount each person needs can vary between 2 and 3 cups each day. Those who are very physically active actually may need more."[65]  Notice the use of the word, "need."  They're not recommending dairy products, they say you *need* them. Their "Cup of Dairy Table" is a long list comprising a variety of milk, yogurt, cheese and milk-based products; and at the bottom of the table is an entry for soymilk.[66] (Maybe the soy lobbyists fought for that little mention; if so, the soda lobbyists will just have to worker harder).

According to the National Institutes of Health, approximately 65% of the human population has a reduced ability to digest lactose after

---

[65] "What foods are included in the Dairy Group?" USDA ChooseMyPlate, https://www.choosemyplate.gov/eathealthy/dairy

[66] Ibid.

infancy.[67] Many other medical findings claim that 75% of the world's population are lactose intolerant.[68]

A large study in Sweden found that women who drank more than 3 glasses of milk per day had nearly double the mortality over 20 years compared to women consuming less than 1 glass per day. And, the heavy milk drinkers had more bone fractures, especially hip fractures.[69] [70]

I still splash a little organic milk in my coffee, but that's it. If you're looking for a dairy replacement for cereal, try unsweetened almond milk. Naturally rich in several vitamins and minerals, especially vitamin E, and low in carbs and calories, it tastes great, doesn't raise blood sugar, and has become the most popular plant milk in the United States.[71]

Humans don't *need* cow's milk. Calves need cow's milk. Assuming you are not a calf, reducing or eliminating dairy products

[67] "Lactose intolerance," MedlinePlus, U.S. National Library of Medicine, NIH. https://ghr.nlm.nih.gov/condition/lactose-intolerance#statistics

[68] "75% of earth population are lactose intolerant: Here's why," choosecompassion.net, Sept. 14, 2017. http://choosecompassion.net/health/75-earth-population-lactose-intolerant-perfectly-natural/

[69] Thomas Campbell, MD, "12 Frightening Facts About Milk," Center for Nutrition Studies (CNS), Updated Oct. 30, 2020. https://nutritionstudies.org/12-frightening-facts-milk/

[70] Krl Michaelsson, lead author, "Milk intake and risk of mortality and fractures in women and men: cohort studies," BMJ 2014;349:g6015, Oct. 28, 2014. https://www.bmj.com/content/349/bmj.g6015

[71] Atli Arnarson, Ph.D., "7 benefits of almond milk," MEDICAL NEWS TODAY, Updated June 2, 2020. https://www.medicalnewstoday.com/articles/318612

can yield many benefits. As to all the hungry calves out there, they should be advised to remain leery of lobbyists.

## Who Likes Cheese?

Everybody! Well, almost everybody. I love cheese. I used to eat cheese twice a day. After discovering the downsides of massive cheese intake, I gradually cut down to once a day, then a few times a week, and eventually once a week. My favorite cheese event is to throw a pizza party! It just makes life fun! And I know I'm spoiled. I grew up in New Jersey, which has the best pizza in America (sorry New York and Chicago, you're good, but not that good).

I'm convinced that the great taste of cheese is amplified wondrously if you make it a treat instead of a staple. No matter how much you love cheese, if you deprive your selfish tastebuds for a few days or a week, it tastes even better.

You should also consider that excessive cheese eating deprives your palate of other delicious endeavors. For example, if you're automatically programmed to buy a brick of cream cheese every time you think about a bagel, stop and look around. You may be surprised to find a great food you can put on a bagel that is even better than a schmear of animal fat. In my own quest to eliminate fatty cream cheese, I discovered that a ripe banana schmeared on a bagel was even richer and tastier than a slab of cream cheese, and much healthier to boot. You can try this at home. Take a fork, and mash a banana onto a toasted bagel slice. It will change your life. At least, it did mine.

(If you really want to go crazy, you can eliminate the bagel, but we'll get into that later). Bananas are a prebiotic food, and good source of fiber, vitamin B6, vitamin C, manganese, potassium and natural antioxidants like dopamine and catechins.[72] A medium banana is a little over 100 calories of mostly carbs so I keep it down to one a day, but marathoners can bump up their banana intake and still stay lean.

We know that diets overloaded with animal fats can lead to heart disease and worse. In addition, for some people, the risk of choking may also be increased. Yes, it's even possible to choke on cheese. According to INJURY FACTS 2017, choking is the fourth leading cause of unintentional injury death.[73] In 2018, 5,084 people died from choking in the United States.[74] While meat of often cited as a prime cause for choking, I was nearly killed by cheese. A few years ago, I was in too much of a rush to attend a seminar at Baruch College in New York. I ducked into a deli, grabbed a bagel and cream cheese, and proceeded to wolf it down in record time. Only it didn't go down. It got stuck. In my throat. I was alone, and extremely lucky that some awkward and barely-informed performance of the Heimlich Maneuver on myself dislodged the bagel/cheese wad that almost killed me. I have since reviewed the correct Heimlich Maneuver, and

---

[72] Adda Bjarnadottir, "11 Evidence-Based Health Benefits of Bananas," HEALTHLINE, Oct. 18, 2018. https://www.healthline.com/nutrition/11-proven-benefits-of-bananas#section1

[73] "Choking Prevention and Rescue Tips," National Safety Council. https://www.nsc.org/home-safety/safety-topics/choking-suffocation

[74] John Elflein, "Number of choking-deaths in the U.S. 1945-2018," STATISTA, Feb. 17, 2020. https://www.statista.com/statistics/527321/deaths-due-to-choking-in-the-us/

so should you.[75]  I can't guarantee that a banana will save your life, but I for one, will take it over a brick of cream cheese any day.

Another great replacement food for cheese is the smooth and creamy, hardly-possible-to-choke-on, *persea americana* aka, avocado.  It's low in sugar, and high in fiber, monounsaturated fatty acids, vitamins B2, B3, B5, B6, C, E, K, folate, potassium, carotenoids such as lutein and zeaxanthin (important for eye health) and antioxidants.[76]  Avocado studies have shown heart healthy and weight loss effects, along with anti-inflammatory, anti-cancer and anti-oxidant properties.[77] [78]

To painlessly reduce your cheese consumption, use the handy, dandy, no-shock-to-the-system CUSTOMIZE YOURSELF gradual cheese-reduction strategy.  Skip a day or two of cheese per week, or knock off 25%.  Return to your 'MORE HARM THAN GOOD LIST,' next to "CHEESE," write down today's date, and your goal,

---

[75] Harrison Lewis, "How to Perform the Heimlich Maneuver on Yourself," wikiHow, Updated Dec. 11, 2020. https://www.wikihow.com/Perform-the-Heimlich-Maneuver-on-Yourself

[76] Adda Bjarnadottir, "Everything you need to know about avocado," MEDICAL NEWS TODAY, Updated Apr. 27, 2020. https://www.medicalnewstoday.com/articles/318620

[77] Mark Dreher, Adrienne Davenport, "Hass Avocado Composition and Potential Health Effects," CRITICAL REVIEWS IN FOOD SCIENCE AND NUTRITION, 2013 May; 53(7): 738-750. https://www.ncbi.nlm.nih.gov/pmc/articles/PMC3664913/

[78] Maha Alkhalaf, lead author, "Anti-oxidant, anti-inflammatory and ant-cancer activities of avocado (Persea americana) fruit and seed extract," JOURNAL OF KING SAUD UNIVERSITY – SCIENCE, Vol. 31, Issue 4, Oct. 2019, pp. 1358-1362. https://www.sciencedirect.com/science/article/pii/S1018364718315714

"25% LESS." Mark your calendar 6 months hence, and it's "25% LEES CHEESE" party time!

## EVOO To The Rescue


Too many Americans and other folks who live away from the Mediterranean perimeter still rely on butter, margarine and the less healthy, cheaper vegetable oils for cooking, schmearing, salad dressings, and the like.  While debates may still rage about the positive and negative nutritional aspects and preferred cooking temperatures of a great variety of vegetable oils, if you wish to take the vegetable oil journey of a thousand miles, consider Lao-tzu's advice about beginning with a first step.  And that first step should be extra virgin olive oil, or as denoted on an increasing number of enlightened restaurant menus, EVOO.

Research presented at the American Heart Association's Prevention, Lifestyle and Cardiometabolic Health Sessions 2020 shows that replacing 5 grams of butter or margarine (about a half of a pat) with the same amount of olive oil was associated with up to a 7% lower risk of coronary artery disease.  With more than 7 grams of olive oil, or a half teaspoon per day, people had a 15% lower risk of cardiovascular disease and a 21% lower risk of coronary artery disease.[79]

---

[79] Sandee LaMotte, "Using olive oil instead of these foods could add years to the life of your heart, study says," CNN HEALTH, Updated Mar. 5, 2020.

The study also made clear that you should not merely add olive oil to your diet. Study author Dr. Frank Hu, Chair of the Department of Nutrition at the Harvard University T. H. Chan School of Public Health said, "The main thing is to replace unhealthy fats with olive oil and that can improve cholesterol, reduce inflammatory biomarkers and improve cardiovascular health."[80]

Non-extra virgin olive oil is fine to use, but extra virgin olive oil has many advantages. EVOO is healthier because it is less refined. EVOO is created solely from pressing, while regular olive oil is derived from combining virgin (pressed) oil and refined (heated or chemically extracted olive oil.[81] EVOO contains fewer chemicals and free radicals than regular olive oil. It's higher in antioxidants than olive oil. And EVOO is full of good fats.[82]

Cooking with olive oil used to have a bad rap. It was rumored that the smoke point/burning point of olive oil would release harmful compounds, but this was proven false by a 2018 Australian study which found that EVOO was even more chemically stable at high

https://www.cnn.com/2020/03/05/health/olive-oil-heart-health-wellness/index.html

[80] Ibid.

[81] Ryan Raman, "Olive Oil vs. Canola Oil: Which Is Healthier?" HEALTHLINE, Updated: May 2, 2019. https://www.healthline.com/nutrition/canola-vs-olive-oil

[82] Gretchen Stelter, "Is extra virgin olive oil better than olive oil?" MEDICAL NEWS TODAY, Updated: July 21, 2020. https://www.medicalnewstoday.com/articles/318397#pure_or_light_virgin_olive_oil

temperatures than other common cooking oils.[83]  Extra virgin olive oil, (but not regular olive oil), produced the lowest levels of trans fats. Coconut oil was second best.  Canola oil was the most unstable, creating more than double the harmful byproducts as EVOO, characterized by the study as exceeding, "the limits permitted for human consumption."[84]

While many excellent extra virgin olive oils are being produced in Spain, Greece, Tunisia and other Mediterranean countries, Italy still leads the pack.  Italian EVOO generally costs more, but I think it's worth it.  I've tasted some great extra virgin olive oils from Spain, Portugal and even California, but overall, I have found that most of the best are from Italy.  In many contests, including the EVOOWR, World Ranking of Extra Virgin Olive Oils 2019, Italy was ranked #1.[85]

For vegetable oil explorers who want to pursue the oil journey of a thousand miles, (while continuing to embrace your favorite EVOO), you can go right past the cheaper, less nutritious, usually genetically

[83] Guillaume De Alzaa, L Ravetti, "Evaluation of Chemical and Physical Changes in Different Commercial Oils during Heating," ACTA SCIENTIFIC NUTRITIONAL HEALTH, Vol. 2, Issue 6, June 2018. https://actascientific.com/ASNH/pdf/ASNH-02-0083.pdf

[84]Ibid. and Sandee LaMotte, "Using olive oil instead of these foods could add years to the life of your heart, study says," CNN HEALTH, Updated Mar. 5, 2020. https://www.cnn.com/2020/03/05/health/olive-oil-heart-health-wellness/index.html

[85] EVOOWR World Ranking of Extra Virgin Olive Oils 2019. http://www.evooworldranking.org/ EN/index.php

modified (GMO) oils like corn, canola[86] and soybean, and follow the food experts who extoll the virtues of the healthy, tasty, albeit more expensive, highly-touted oils like avocado, coconut, hempseed, walnut, a variety of infused-oils, and other contenders fighting for market shelf space while rotating in and out of vogue. It's an expanding field for a new wave of oil connoisseurs, with passions rivaling those of wine connoisseurs.

---

[86] Over 90% of the canola crops grown in the United States are GMO. Jillian Kubala, "Is Canola Oil Healthy? All You Need to Know, HEALTHLINE, Feb. 7, 2019. https://www.healthline.com/nutrition/is-canola-oil-healthy
And Meredith Schafer, lead author, "The Establishment of Genetically Engineered Canola Populations in the U.S.," PLOS ONE, Oct. 5, 2011. https://www.ncbi.nlm.nih.gov/pmc/articles/PMC3187797/

# How I Broke Butter's Heart But Saved Mine

Not only did I used to eat cheese twice a day, but I also averaged about twice a day for butter too. Looking back and estimating, I consumed approximately one stick of butter per week, or 52 sticks a year, which equals 13 pounds a year, or 130 pounds in ten years. Since I ate butter for almost 40 years, that's around 520 pounds, or about one-quarter of a ton of butter. So what's your butter tonnage?

Now, if you add a few tons of cheese and meat to that rough equation, you might be able to hear your arteries screaming for a Jewish deli owner's cardiologist son or daughter[87] to save you, but since arteries don't generally scream out loud, you might be out of luck.

If you've ever been to Paris, and stepped into any boulangerie for baguette and butter, (and don't even try to ask for it in English, because odds are they'll look at you like you're from Mars even if they speak perfect English), you've scored one of the most incredible taste sensations on Earth. And if you've had any other great bread

---

[87] As of 2016, only 13% of adult cardiologists in the United States were women, but as of 2019, cardiology fellowships for women were up to 21.5%. Laxmi Mehta, lead author, "Current Demographic Status of Cardiologists in the United States," JAMA Cardiology, Sept. 11, 2019.
https://www.ncbi.nlm.nih.gov/pmc/articles/PMC6739735/

with butter anywhere else, you may have come close. Either way, it would be totally understandable if you swore to never give up eating bread and butter. To be honest, I'd recommend to anyone going to Paris, seek baguette and butter first, and then think about visiting the Louvre or Musee de l'Orangerie.

I won't try persuade you to give up butter, although doing so may yield considerable benefits, but I can tell that you that it's possible to not butter your bread, ever, and still have a wonderful life. It's as simple as finding a great tasting extra virgin olive oil, dipping in your favorite bread or roll, savoring it, and then repeating the experience until you admit that you can live without butter.

After recognizing that I was just as happy with a tasty EVOO as with butter, and realizing that I did not need butter as a backup for the cream cheese I was no longer consuming, I harked back to my last trip down the supermarket chips aisle when I just pushed my cart past the chips, and kept going, forever, into the sunset (or maybe it was the fish department), and did the same thing in the dairy section. I rolled past the sticks and stacks and bricks and tubs of butter, and just kept going, to the same tune,

*Walk on by (don't stop)*...
*Walk on by (don't stop)*...[88]

That was more than 20 years ago, and I don't miss butter at all. Not a bit. I can live without it. I can live longer without it. I know

---

[88] Dionne Warwick. "Walk On By." *Make Way for Dionne Warwick.* Scepter. 1964.

that if I'm in a restaurant, I may unwittingly wind up with a dish of something cooked with butter. On rare occasion, I may even butter a roll if their olive oil is awful or missing in action. And if I want to, I can watch CASABLANCA, because... I'll always have Paris.

# The French Paradox

The French paradox is an observation advanced by French epidemiologists[89] that recognizes France's low coronary heart disease death rates despite a high intake of animal fats. Since then, many explanations for this phenomena have been proven inconclusive, incomplete or incorrect. It's worth mentioning that many studies have concluded that moderate, regular drinking of red wine leads to lower mortality from heart disease. And, red wine accomplishes this feat while an equivalent consumption of beer or hard liquor does not.[90] They also present evidence that the practice of "binge" drinking, which is more popular in the United States and in many Northern European countries than in France, is associated with increased rates of heart disease.[91] Here again, we should also consider the benefits of the Mediterranean diet, rich in vegetables and fruits including

[89] Richard JL, Cambien F, Ducimetière P., "Epidemiologic characteristics of coronary disease in France," Nouv Presse Med 1981;10:1111–4.

[90] Gronbaek M, Becker U, Johansen D, et al. Type of alcohol consumed and mortality from all causes, coronary heart disease, and cancer. Ann Intern Med 2000;133:411–9.

[91] Jean Ferrieres, "The French paradox: lessons for other countries," HEART, 2004 Jan; 90(1): 107-111.
https://www.ncbi.nlm.nih.gov/pmc/articles/PMC1768013/

grapes. We'll get more into red wine and resveratrol later, but for now, let's just say that if you've adopted anything close to a Mediterranean diet and/or already made some significant reductions in animal fat intake, and for good measure, your total cholesterol is close to 150 mg/dL, it's fair to assume that a little butter won't kill you.

I might add that most of my life has been spent in the world of cinema, where among other things, I've curated Arthouse Film Festival for 29 years. Among the million questions I get asked whenever I show my in face in public is, "What's your favorite movie?" It pains me to admit that I cannot answer this question because there are at least 100 films tied for first on my list, and about another 500 movies I feel guilty about not including; and then I can't help feeling like an idiot whenever I try to explain it. But for those of you who may not die from eating butter, I'll mention one movie. DIVA (1981) is a mesmerizing, French thriller which may not directly address the French paradox, but it just happens to make baguette and butter utterly irresistible. Directed by Jean-Jacques Beineix, starring Wilhelmenia Fernandez, DIVA is a hugely entertaining, surprisingly instructive, unforgettable masterwork that deserves at least 100 pages of raves and analysis, but I will refer here to just one scene. That scene involves an obsessive character showing another how to butter a baguette. That's it. That's all I'm going to say. You'll have to see the movie.

Bottom line, if you're committed to butter, and you want to cut down, you should probably avoid seeing DIVA. Also, stick with grass-fed butter. Then use the same CUSTOMIZE YOURSELF approach that you have applied to fried foods, meat and cheese. On

your 'MORE HARM THAN GOOD LIST,' next to "BUTTER,"
write down today's date, and your goal, "25% LESS." Then, mark
down a 6 month "25% LESS BUTTER" celebration on your party
calendar!

# One More Hat Tip To The Mediterranean Way

While many good diets are plant-based and eliminate animal products altogether, the very popular and healthy Mediterranean diet does not completely eliminate meat and dairy. It recommends eating more fruits and vegetables, aiming for seven to ten servings a day; opting for whole grains like bulgur and farro; relying on extra virgin olive oil as a replacement for butter; increasing seafood consumption, twice a week or more, grilling instead of frying; and decreasing salt, replacing it with herbs and spices. Meat should be reduced, with smaller portions, and substitutions with fish, poultry or beans. Dairy is acceptable as Greek or plain yogurt, and small amounts of a variety of cheeses.[92]

My mother's, *The key is moderation* dovetails very nicely with the Mediterranean diet. If you're looking for a dietary direction, go the Mediterranean way. (For people with high cardiovascular risk, I refer you to a large study published in THE NEW ENGLAND JOURNAL

---

[92] Mayo Clinic Staff, "Mediterranean diet: A heart-healthy eating plan," MAYO CLINIC, June 21, 2019. https://www.mayoclinic.org/healthy-lifestyle/nutrition-and-healthy-eating/in-depth/mediterranean-diet/art-20047801

OF MEDICINE.[93]   It concluded that participants assigned to a Mediterranean diet supplemented with extra virgin olive oil or nuts had fewer major cardiovascular events than those assigned to a reduced fat diet).

My own personal, customized plan has eliminated meat and poultry altogether, and while not in perfect synch with the Mediterranean diet, it has much in common.  Again, I raise this to emphasize that you should think about the changes you might like to make, observe and pay attention to your own physical reactions, experiment and evolve your own custom plan, and be confident that it eventually will become the safest, most enjoyable, sustainable plan you can achieve.

---

[93] Ramon Estruch, lead author, "Primary Prevention of Cardiovascular Disease with a Mediterranean Diet Supplemented with Extra-Virgin Olive or Nuts," NEW ENGLAND JOURNAL OF MEDICINE, Updated: June 21, 2018. https://www.nejm.org/doi/10.1056/NEJMoa1800389

# Part II: *Plants And More Plants*

# The Big Salad

*You know, if it was a regular salad, I wouldn't have said anything,*
*but you had to have the BIG SALAD!*
*-George Costanza*[94]

Somehow, as I weaned myself off fatty meats and fried foods, I
was fortunate to develop a wild passion for salads. Big salads. Big
salads with lots of everything in them. I try to eat a big salad every
day. If I miss a day, I can't wait to make the next big salad. If a
restaurant doesn't offer a really good salad, I will avoid that
establishment. If you have a passion for big salads, or even medium-
size salads, you know what I'm talking about.

I'd rather not preach the particulars of the ultimate big salad, but
you can enjoy the benefits of your own customized salad simply by
collecting a small mountain of your favorite ingredients, and grabbing
a big knife. It's really easy, and fun. Just don't cut off any fingers.

In general, with all of your vegetables, the more colorful, the
better. Stick with leafy greens, avoid iceberg lettuce, and feel free to
experiment a lot. I stock an ample battery of nuts, seeds, herbs and

---

[94] George Costanza (Jason Alexander), "The Big Salad." *Seinfeld,* Season 6,
Episode 2, NBC, Sept. 29,1994.

91

an alternating array of seafood to pump up the protein. If legumes are your thing, throw 'em in the bowl. You're only limited by your imagination.

Caveat emptor #1 with all salads relates to the almost universal, shocking awfulness of bottled salad dressings. We'll cover more of the life-saving benefits of reading labels as we go on, but for now, just pick up almost any bottle of store-bought salad dressing, and read the ingredients. You may be repulsed. It's doubtful, you'll be turned on. Genetically modified organisms (GMOs), inferior vegetable oils, high-fructose corn syrup, trans fats, Monosodium glutamate (MSG), excessive salt and sugar, gums, dyes, additives, unpronounceable chemicals and plenty of other stuff that you can live without are commonly found inside these vessels. What passes as balsamic vinegar in some commercial brands is actually white vinegar with added coloring, sugars and thickening agents.[95] The fat and calorie contents of many creamy varieties are off the charts. Don't hamper or destroy the nutritional value of your fantastic, customized salad with the questionable contents of a crappy bottled salad dressing.

It's not impossible to find a healthy, bottled salad dressing that may happen to deserve the much abused "natural" moniker, or better yet, organic, but the best alternative is simply to rely on extra-virgin olive oil along with the best balsamic vinegar you can afford.

---

[95] Molly Carter, "5 Salad Ingredients That Are Actually Killing Your Diet," THE PATH. http://www.thepathmag.com/5-salad-ingredients-that-are-actually-killing-your-diet/

According to Harvard's Dr. Hu, just switching to olive oil and vinegar, "can have significant health benefits in the long run."[96]

Balsamic vinegar connoisseurs focus on two Italian regions, Modena and Reggio Emilia. The finest examples are slow cooked, then aged in barrels for between 12 and 25 years.[97] They're thick, tasty and can easily cost $200 or more. The more affordable "IGP" varieties are produced and aged in these regions, but the grapes may come from another region. Many are in the $10 to $30 range, which may still sound expensive, but when you consider that you only pour a small amount at a time, and how quickly you can drain a bottle of commercial salad dressing, purchasing a great balsamic vinegar is a pretty good deal. It's also a worthy vehicle to invest your savings from not buying french fries.

If you haven't done it before, just think about the wonders of making your own customized salad dressing. You are free to experiment, and invent something terrific in a matter of minutes. My own salad dressing journey continues to evolve. Whether a medium salad-eater, or a radical EVOO aficionado, I present to you my latest incarnation.

You'll need fresh basil for this. Without fresh basil, your life will never be complete. Besides the irresistible, aromatic deliciousness,

[96] Sandee LaMotte, "Using olive oil instead of these foods could add years to the life of your heart, study says," CNN HEALTH, Updated Mar. 5, 2020. https://www.cnn.com/2020/03/05/health/olive-oil-heart-health-wellness/index.html

[97] Nikhita Venugopal, "The Best Balsamic Vinegars, According to People Who Use a Lot of It," NEW YORK, Apr. 12, 2019. https://nymag.com/strategist/article/best-balsamic-vinegar-brands.html

vitamin K-loaded basil has been found to exhibit antimicrobial, anti-inflammatory, antioxidant and anti-cancer activity.[98]

*THE BIG SALAD DRESSING*
*Extra virgin olive oil*
*Balsamic vinegar*
*Dijon mustard*
*Basil (5-10 fresh leaves)*
*Oregano (6-8 fresh leaves, or 2 pinches of dry oregano)*
*Garlic (1 small, minced garlic clove, or a pinch of dry garlic)*
*Turmeric (2-3 pinches)*
*Fresh ground pepper*

**1)** Take a small, shallow mixing bowl, and plop in a generous spoonful of your favorite Dijon mustard, (you can experiment here too, with a great range of Dijon mustards, from mild to very spicy). Add a dribble of that fantastic balsamic vinegar you paid too much for. Then, use a fork to lightly and rapidly whip/whisk/swirl until you have a creamy consistency.

**2)** Pour in a short shot (one or two tablespoons) of EVOO, and whip/whisk/swirl some more until you again attain the same level of creaminess. Optional: at this point, you may or may not want to add a another shot of EVOO, and fork-whip it some more.

---

[98] Spezzatino Magazine, "What's so healthy about basil?" Precision Nutrition. https://www.precisionnutrition.com/healthy-basil

**3)** Depending on how much you love fresh basil and how much fresh basil you have, wash and dry 5 to 10 leaves, and tear up half of them. Spread them on the creamy surface, and mash them lightly with your fork. Then, take the other half of your basil leaves and do the same.

**4)** Theoretically, you could quit here, declare victory, and mix it into your salad. Better to opt for some herbs and spices. Fresh oregano is awesome, but you can use the dried variety if that's all you have. Add a smidge of mashed garlic or sprinkle of garlic powder. (I go very light with the garlic only because while I like garlic, I've learned that garlic doesn't like me. Many claims have been made about the health benefits of garlic, and while it has impressed in the test tube,[99] conclusive evidence awaits further study.[100] I am convinced that the perfect amount of garlic is just enough to keep away vampires). Tighten the screw on your pepper mill, and turn the crank one half rotation (or if you're a pepper fiend, a little more). Last but not least, you can load in a blizzard of turmeric. I go crazy with the turmeric, but you may dial it up or down to your taste. (If a fraction of the health claims made for turmeric are true, this will add years to your life). A couple of light stirs and you're done.

**5)** Toss maniacally into your big salad, and savor Nirvana, (the transcendent state of perfect peace and happiness, like heaven or the

---

[99] "6 Surprising Ways Garlic Boosts Your Health," Cleveland Clinic, Dec. 7, 2020. https://health.clevelandclinic.org/6-surprising-ways-garlic-boosts-your-health/

[100] Leyla Bayan, Peir Koulivand, Ali Gorji, "Garlic: a review of potential therapeutic effects," AVICENNA JOURNAL OF PHYTOMEDICINE, 2014 Jan-Feb; 4(1): 1-14. https://www.ncbi.nlm.nih.gov/pmc/articles/PMC4103721/

final goal of Buddhism, or the grunge-version, fronted by Kurt Cobain, your choice).

# Grain Wars

Many of the current crop of best-selling books about nutrition, health and longevity advocate for the total elimination of grains in everyone's diet. A few settle for massive reduction. Their authors present an extensive array of compelling data and associations to support their assertions. They argue that grains typically have high levels of starch and gluten, undesirable additives and chemicals, cause blood pressure spikes, and can increase insulin to levels which can lead to diabetes, heart disease, cancer, dementia and Alzheimer's. They point out that modern grains are often drenched with glyphosate, (an herbicide that can increase cancer risks by 41% according to a lengthy University of Washington study published in the journal MUTATION in 2019).[101] [102] [103]

---

[101] Emily Dixon, "Common weed killer glyphosate increases cancer risk by 41%, study says," CNN HEALTH, Feb. 15, 2019.
https://www.cnn.com/2019/02/14/health/us-glyphosate-cancer-study-scli-intl/index.html

[102] Luoping Zhang, lead author, "Exposure to glyphosate-based herbicides and risk for non-Hodgkin lymphoma: A meta-analysis and supporting evidence," MUTATION RESEARCH, Vol. 781, July-Sept. 2019, pp. 186-206.
https://www.sciencedirect.com/science/article/pii/S1383574218300887

[103] Jackson Holtz, "UW study: Exposure to chemical in Roundup increases risk for cancer," UW NEWS, Feb. 13, 2019.

Wheat is their biggest enemy, but rye, oats, semolina, spelt and barley are also offenders. Many of them damn gluten-free starches like corn and quinoa, while some allow them. Soy has its friends and enemies. Buckwheat is mostly accepted. The grain fighters condemn bread, cereal, pasta, pizza, pastries, crackers, cookies and beer. I would bet that many of these authors' most fervent followers will get about as close to a toasted bagel as a coiled rattlesnake.

A number of the grain warriors say to avoid gluten entirely. And for a portion of the population, this can be a lifesaving advice. More than 300,000 people in the United States (about 1%) have celiac disease. They cannot tolerate even a tiny amount of gluten. Many other people have gluten sensitivity. Celiac disease can be identified with a blood test, so no one should be guessing about whether they are afflicted.[104]

Supermarkets have responded by offering a colossal range of gluten-free foods. Restaurants pack their menus with gluten-free choices. Many people have been convinced that gluten-free diets promote weight loss, boost energy, treat autism or just make them feel better. But before going gluten-free, it is highly recommended to first see a doctor. Once a person has avoided gluten for an extended period

https://www.washington.edu/news/2019/02/13/uw-study-exposure-to-chemical-in-roundup-increases-risk-for-cancer/

[104] Holly Strawbridge, "Going gluten-free just because? Here's what you need to know," HARVARD HEALTH, Updated: Jan. 29, 2020. https://www.health.harvard.edu/blog/going-gluten-free-just-because-heres-what-you-need-to-know-201302205916

of time, it can become difficult to determine if celiac disease or gluten sensitivity may be present.[105]

It is important to note that gluten-free diets can cause nutritional deficiencies, presenting a variety of challenges. Also, gluten is commonly contained in many other not-so-obvious products including sauces, flavorings, roasted nuts, soups, couscous, matzo, some medications, and even toothpaste. Abandoning wheat and other common grains can cause deficiencies of dietary fiber and vitamins. Fortified breads and cereals are common in the United States, often serving as a major source of B vitamins.[106] Care should to be taken to replace missing fiber and vitamins by consuming more fruits, vegetables, gluten-free whole grains like buckwheat (but not buckwheat flour) and quinoa, and beans (although beans have their detractors too). Consider that gluten-free cookies and desserts are still cookies and desserts. Also, many gluten-free products have added cornstarch, rice starch, potato starch and tapioca starch. These are carbohydrates with high glycemic indexes (GI), often as high as wheat products, which may be OK for marathon runners, but not so good for people with diabetic issues.[107] It's probably best to avoid these added starches altogether.

If you are not suffering from obesity, diabetes, high blood pressure, heart disease or some other serious malady, ask yourself

---

[105] Ibid.

[106] Ibid.

[107] "Glycemic index for 60+ foods," HARVARD HEALTH, Updated: Jan. 6, 2020. https://www.health.harvard.edu/diseases-and-conditions/glycemic-index-and-glycemic-load-for-100-foods

why you would want to make such radical changes in your diet, and how you plan to address the new challenges of finding, liking (and being liked by) a number of replacement/substitution foods. Also, don't forget that somewhere around 95% of dieters don't stick to a new diet for more than a year. And, you could also ask yourself, is death by bagel the worst way to go? (If you find yourself mashing a banana onto your hand instead of a bagel, you have your answer).

It's here that I suggest you apply the common-sense, slow-and-steady-wins-the-game, gradual, CUSTOMIZE YOURSELF reduction approach. Perhaps, lower your gluten to start. Try eating less bread. See how it feels. Get comfortable with it, then you may want to consider avoiding gluten, and to what extent. Be prepared to substitute with gluten-free whole grains. Seek out a buckwheat pizza. Swap some bread and rolls for sweet potatoes, preferably not fried. Try baked. Try boiled. Add other fiber-rich vegetables and fruits. Experiment. Check out new foods. Customize!

And for those of you who are convinced that your current gluten consumption is just fine for you, I'll share 1 anecdote. Even at 110 years old, my mother is not satisfied without having at least 2 loaves of whole wheat and 2 loaves of rye bread in her freezer at all times. I dare any grain warrior to try and talk her out it.

In my own case, I have gradually reduced my bread/rolls/cookie intake by about 50%. Over that stretch, I dropped a few pounds, (not that I needed to), and generally felt slightly better overall. Nothing significant to report, I'm not waving a flag for the grain fighters, but if they can steer their adherents towards more healthful habits, and withstand baguette-wielding Parisians, c'est la vie. In the foreseeable future, as I get comfortable with a few more whole grain and vegetable substitutes, I may head for 75%, (and throw a few more parties for myself). It's worth repeating, my customized grain plan is for me, not for everybody. With some reasonable thought and effort, and a little patience and creativity, you will refine, improve and CUSTOMIZE YOURSELF.

## A Short Quiz

It's an easy quiz.

You will not be graded on a curve.

It's a pass/fail quiz.

If you fail, you die.

This quiz will test your knowledge of the effects of cocaine, methamphetamine and other life-threatening substances.

Ready?

--Question #1: Name a drug, food or other substance that can not only be a substitute to addictive drugs like cocaine, but can be even more rewarding and attractive.[108]

--Answer #1: _____

--Question #2: Name a substance as addictive as cocaine or methamphetamine that can cause similar withdrawal symptoms

---

[108] Magalie Lenoir, lead author, "Intense Sweetness Surpasses Cocaine Reward," PLOS ONE, Aug. 1, 2007.
https://journals.plos.org/plosone/article?id=10.1371/journal.pone.0000698

including headache, dizziness, nausea, fatigue, anxiety, restlessness, sleeping problems, cravings and depression.[109] [110]

--Answer #2: _____


--Question #3: Besides cocaine and methamphetamine, name a substance that causes gum disease and tooth decay, and can cause seizures and heart disease.[111]

--Answer #3: _____


If you answered, "sugar" to all three questions, you passed the quiz. If you failed the quiz, you may not die right away, but excessive sugar consumption could easily hasten your death.

---

[109] Adrienne Santos-Longhurst, "What Is a Sugar Detox? Effects and How to Avoid Sugar," HEALTHLINE, Updated: Aug. 20, 2020.
https://www.healthline.com/health/sugar-detox-symptoms#beating-side-effects

[110] Sara Lindberg, Erin Kelly, "Your Anxiety Loves Sugar. Eat These 3 Things Instead," HEALTHLINE, June 23, 2020.
https://www.healthline.com/health/mental-health/how-sugar-harms-mental-health#highsand-lows

[111] R. Alan Leo, "Unraveling the secrets of the epilepsy diet," THE HARVARD GAZETTE, May 24, 2012.
https://news.harvard.edu/gazette/story/2012/05/unraveling-the-secrets-of-the-epilepsy-diet/

## Sugar Or Cocaine, Which Is Worse For You?

As with cocaine, many researchers have concluded that sugar is one of the most addictive substances known to humankind. A study at Connecticut College demonstrated that Oreos are just as addictive as cocaine, at least for lab rats.[112]

It's doubtful that many of you will wake up tomorrow, and pick up a bag of sugar in one hand and a bag of cocaine in the other, and wonder, "Hmmm, which one should I choose?" For those of you who may face that decision, my guess is, you'll choose both.

It's fair to say that cocaine consumption is limited in many places because it is very expensive and illegal. Penalties for possession and sale are quite severe. You can buy massive quantities of cheap sugar everywhere, consume it at home or in public, and be confident that you won't get thrown in jail for scarfing sweets. The law definitely discourages consumption of powdered cocaine and crack, but not sugar. The sugar industry and the food industries that support it are strong business forces, and have the overwhelming support of their addicted consumers, (similar to cocaine adherents).

---

[112] Connecticut College, "Are Oreos addictive? Research says yes," SCIENCE DAILY, Oct. 15, 2013.
https://www.sciencedaily.com/releases/2013/10/131015123341.htm

In 2012, as mayor of New York City, Michael Bloomberg tried to limit the sales of sugary drinks larger than 16 ounces, and the cries of outrage were spine rattling. Jon Stewart wailed injustice on the DAILY SHOW, going so far as to play a Fox News clip, proclaiming, "I agree with Tucker Carlson, Tucker Carlson is right, and I will never forgive you for that, Michael Bloomberg."[113] Amazing! Jon Stewart agreed with Tucker Carlson! Two years later, Judge Eugene F. Pigott Jr. of the New York State Court of Appeals, the highest court in the state, wrote a 20 page opinion rejecting Bloomberg's attempt to regulate sugar intake by the good citizens of New York.[114] Mission accomplished, a few months later, Jon Stewart retired to a farm in New Jersey to raise goats and drink soda.

Setting aside the popular support for keeping sugar incredibly cheap and widely available, both cocaine and sugar are clearly bad for you, but which one is worse?

Cocaine is a vasoconstrictor that makes your heart pump faster while narrowing your blood vessels, placing additional strain on your heart muscles, which can lead to heart attack. It also increases the risk of atherosclerosis, hardening and thickening your arteries.[115] At

---

[113] Christine Friar, "Jon Stewart Criticizes Bloomberg's New York Soda Ban," HUFFPOST, Updated: Aug. 1, 2012. https://www.huffpost.com/entry/jon-stewart-bloomberg-soda-ban-video_n_1562011

[114] Michael Grynbaum, "New York's Ban on Sodas Is Rejected by Final Court," THE NEW YORK TIMES, June 26, 2014. https://www.nytimes.com/2014/06/27/nyregion/city-loses-final-appeal-on-limiting-sales-of-large-sodas.html

[115] Chris D'Alessandro, "Cocaine might be bad for your heart, but sugar is so much worse," ROOSTER, July 18, 2018. https://therooster.com/blog/cocaine-might-be-bad-you-sugar-takes-cake

least, cocaine won't make you fat. Sugar causes inflammation,[116] [117] shrinks your brain,[118] [119] and leads to obesity, which increases the risks of heart disease, stroke, type 2 diabetes and some cancers. And, as sugar makes you fatter, it also increases your craving for sugar.[120]

You can choose to do cocaine. You need the money to pay for it, an accessible and reliable drug dealer, and a special tolerance for the legal risks involved. It's really challenging to choose to *not* do sugar. Just about every food product sold in a box, bag, can, jar, pouch or wrapper has added sugar. You really have to be a diligent detective to avoid added sugar.

While it's more challenging to study the effects of cocaine on its users, sugar studies abound. According to one Cleveland Clinic study, men and women who consumed one or more sugar-sweetened

---

[116] Jessica Caporuscio, "Does sugar cause inflammation in the body?" MEDICAL NEWS TODAY, Sept. 19, 2019. https://www.medicalnewstoday.com/articles/326386

[117] Mary Jane Brown, Ph.D., "Does Sugar Cause Inflammation in the Body?" HEALTHLINE, Nov. 12, 2017. https://www.healthline.com/nutrition/sugar-and-inflammation

[118] Stephen Luntz, "Sugar Shrinks the Brain," AUSTRALIAN SCIENCE, Nov. 2012. http://www.australasianscience.com.au/article/issue-november-2012/sugar-shrinks-brain.html

[119] Karen Peart, "The effect of sugar on the brain? Glucose rush shrinks brain cell powerhouse," YALE NEWS, Feb. 25, 2016. https://news.yale.edu/2016/02/25/sugar-rush-shrinks-brain-cell-powerhouse

[120] Chris D'Alessandro, "Cocaine might be bad for your heart, but sugar is so much worse," ROOSTER, July 18, 2018. https://therooster.com/blog/cocaine-might-be-bad-you-sugar-takes-cake

sodas a day had a higher risk of stroke.[121]   A Harvard School of Public Health study linked approximately 180,000 deaths a year worldwide to sugary drink consumption.[122] [123]   Cocaine would have to get a lot cheaper to cause that many annual deaths.

So, which is worse?  I'll leave that up to you, or you can follow the path of the MYSTIC MAN, Peter Tosh,

*I don't sniff them cocaine*
*Choke brain…*
*I man don't*
*Drink pink, blue, yellow, green soda…*
*'Cause I'm a man of the past*
*And I'm livin' in the present*
*And I'm walking in the future*
*Stepping in the future*[124]

---

[121] Live Science Staff, "Daily Soda Consumption Increases Stroke Risk," LIVESCIENCE, May 30, 2013. https://www.livescience.com/36272-soda-consumption-stroke-risk.html

[122] Michael Winter, "Study links 180,000 global deaths to sugary drinks," USA TODAY, Mar. 19, 2013. https://www.usatoday.com/story/news/nation/2013/03/19/sugary-drinks-deaths-research/2001191/?csp=Dailybriefing

[123] Live Science Staff, "Daily Soda Consumption Increases Stroke Risk," LIVE SCIENCE, May 30, 2013. https://www.livescience.com/28040-sugar-sweetened-beverages-deaths.html

[124] Peter Tosh. *Mystic Man*. Rolling Stones Records. 1979.

# Sugar Or Cocaine, Which Is More Profitable?

According to the Rand Corporation, estimated cocaine spending from 2006 to 2016 fell by 59% to a piddling $23 billion in the world's biggest cocaine market, the United States of America.[125] [126] Presently, the global sugar market is heading towards a not-too-shabby $100 billion annual haul.[127] Add the multiplier effects of all the food industries using sugar products to increase their sales and profit margins, and the sugary foods biz is humongous.

For coke dealers, supply chains are unstable, transportation is challenging, competition is murderous (literally), legal risks are enormous, and demand is uneven. Profits are high, but so is the stress.

---

[125] Jason Sullum, "Americans Spend Nearly As Much on Illegal Drugs As They Do on Booze, Which Shows What a Ripoff Prohibition Is," REASON, Aug. 20, 2019. https://reason.com/2019/08/20/americans-spend-nearly-as-much-on-illegal-drugs-as-they-do-on-booze-which-shows-what-a-ripoff-prohibition-is/

[126] Beau Kilmer, lead author, "How Big Is the U.S. Market for Illegal Drugs?" THE RAND CORPORATION, 2014. https://www.rand.org/content/dam/rand/pubs/research_briefs/RB9700/RB9770/RAND_RB9770.pdf

[127] "Sugar Market Nears $90 Billion by 2024 – Analysis by Type, Application, and Geography – ResearchAndMarkets.com, BUSINESSWIRE, Aug. 29, 2019. https://www.businesswire.com/news/home/20190829005286/en/Sugar-Market-Nears-90-Billion-2024--

Sugar dealers have more customers, lower risks, many friends in Washington, great marketing, and booming sales. Profits are reliable, and their competition employs fewer mercenaries who are out to kill them.

Neither drug dealers nor sugar dealers seem to care much about the medical, social or economic costs (wasted resources, reduced work output and the like) incurred by their customers. The United States government has spent well over a $1 trillion since President Nixon launched the 'war on drugs.'[128] Our health care system has spent many more trillions of dollars dealing with soaring obesity, diabetes and heart disease rates, and other problems caused by excessive sugar consumption.

Who pays?

We do.

I have two suggestions:

**#1)** Show drug dealers, who are quite experienced at selling unhealthy products to a highly-addicted consumer base, the data on how much money is being made by the very low risk, legal, sugary food industries. Maybe some of them will drop their stress-inducing, illegal drug operations in favor of adopting a proven, dynamic business model which boasts legal and safer methods to sell a different product to a much larger population of highly-addicted consumers. Then, when the increased competition in all the sugar-related industries gets too fierce, the business will suffer, the violent

---

[128] Betsy Pearl, "Ending the War on Drugs: By the Numbers," CENTER FOR AMERICAN PROGRESS, June 27, 2018.
https://www.americanprogress.org/issues/criminal-justice/reports/2018/06/27/452819/ending-war-drugs-numbers/

players will start killing each other, and some of the ex-drug dealers will turn to selling products less harmful than sugar. (I know, it's a stretch).

Or,

**#2)** Consume less sugar.

How much less? Consider that 200 years ago, the average American ate 2 pounds of sugar a year. By 1970, that increased to 123 pounds of sugar. Nowadays, estimates range from 152 - 180 pounds of sugar per person each year.[129] [130]

Consume how much less sugar?

A lot less.

---

[129] "How Much Sugar Do You Eat? You May Be Surprised!" dhhs.nh.gov
https://www.dhhs.nh.gov/dphs/nhp/documents/sugar.pdf

[130] Gerald Curatola, DDS, "How much sugar does the average person consume every year?" SHARECARE.
https://www.sharecare.com/health/carbohydrates/sugar-consume-every-year

# Sugar Is A Recreational Drug

If the unconditional love you feel by staring into your dog's eyes and promising that you will never feed him french fries, (and therefore you have forsaken them too), is your mantra, you can certainly apply that logic to a donut, or any other blob of sugar and fat. Admittedly, trying to convince anyone (except Homer Simpson) that they're addicted to sugary food products, and doomed to suffer grave consequences unless they stop the madness is a worthy endeavor, but frankly, a hard sell. Sugar has a colossal reputation as being the great reward, an irresistible treat, the star of the show, a guaranteed draw to get people together and have fun! Come on, you're invited to a party! You don't wanna miss it! We're gonna have cake!

If one accepts that sugar is a recreational drug, it may be easier to balance logic with desire. Let the gradual, one-step-at-a-time, practical CUSTOMIZE YOURSELF approach be your guide. The goal of a 25% reduction in sugar intake is your first step.

Let's examine the process of consuming a dessert. How long does it take you to polish off a dessert? Ice cream usually takes longer than cake. Ice cream in a cone takes more time to ingest than with a dish and spoon. Cake, unless you're a maniac with a fork, takes longer to eat than cookies. Pie is pretty close to cake, although a tangy berry might slow you down. Cookies are a wild card. It's really easy to unconsciously obliterate a pile of cookies and not even notice until you're pawing around for crumbs.

Try timing yourself eating a big cookie. How long does it take? Two minutes? Three minutes? Pretty quick, huh? Was it worth it? What about 2 big cookies? Does it take twice as long, or do you slow down for the second one? How much walking or running will it take to burn off those 2 giant cookies? Mind you, if you don't burn it off, it will remain as fat. And if you look in the mirror, you will see where that new fat is, and you will wish that it wasn't there. Guilt. Shame. Oh, the agony.

It's time for moderation (like Mom said). Whatever your dessert/treat/sugar intake is now, take stock of it, measure it, be aware of it, and make a simple, gradual plan to reduce it by 25%. If you are a cookie monster, it's easy to count up the cookies you're eating. Don't cheat. You know how many you're eating. Whether you're eating 8 cookies a day, or 8 cookies a month, starting today, reduce your intake by 25%. That's it. That's all you have to do. You're done. You know you can do it.

Let's say you're a 4-cookies-at-a-time user. OK, now make it 3. You've only subtracted 1 cookie. One lousy cookie. No big deal. Instead of spending 8 minutes consuming cookies, you'll do it for 6 minutes. If you save 2 minutes a day for a year, that's 730 minutes a year. You've just created more than 12 hours of free time. Now you can stop complaining about how you never have enough time for yourself.

Or, if you like, you can slow down a little, and really savor those precious cookies, really enjoy them like you've never done before. Turn off the television. Really focus on those delicious cookies. I bet they taste even better, and now you're back to 8 minutes of cookie eating, or maybe even longer. So you see, it's possible to *extend* your cookie eating time, and eat *fewer* cookies, and enjoy them even more!

Think of eating 1 less cookie a day as eating 365 less cookies a year. In 10 years, that's 3,650 cookies that you didn't eat. Visualize that Mount Everest of cookies which is in front of you, instead of inside you. Now look in the mirror. Wow, you look mahvelous! And you feel better too! Think of all the money you saved on those ridiculously overpriced cookies. Soon, you will be able to buy that sports car you've always dreamed about. What color will you choose?

Look at the big picture, if eating fewer cookies makes you live longer, you can eat more cookies when you're old and still alive than when you're dead. Right? Be strong! It's only 1 cookie. And you'll be a big success! You don't have to give up cookies. Just the 1. In a couple of days, you won't even miss it. You'll be laughing about how silly it was to think that it was even a challenge. But you should also be proud that you achieved something healthy. A tiny sacrifice made you a better person. In fact, you never have to make another cookie sacrifice again. You can maintain your present, reasonable, comfortable, slightly-reduced cookie consumption for the rest of your life! And be better for it! Congratulations!

Now, on your 'MORE HARM THAN GOOD LIST,' next to "COOKIES," write down today's date, and your goal, "25% LESS." Next, mark on you calendar, 6 months from today,"25% FEWER COOKIES" to throw yourself another party (you can skip the cake). Give yourself a pat on the back. (It should be easier to reach your back now that you're eating fewer cookies). You don't have to further reduce your cookie consumption at all, but on this wonderful anniversary celebration day, just think about maybe eating 1 less cookie. You don't have to do it. It's totally optional. Just think about it. If you decide to further reduce your cookie intake on your fabulous 6 month anniversary, you only have 1 more thing to do. Make a note on your calendar 6 months in the future to throw yourself a "50% FEWER COOKIES" party!

# 'Scuse Me While I Miss The Pie

From show to show, Jimi Hendrix often changed the lyrics in his songs just for the hell of it. "'Scuse me while I miss the pie" could have been the most famous line in PURPLE HAZE.[131] With all the guitar distortion and feedback, it's hard to tell. You'll just have to listen to it yourself and decide. Anyway, pie is great, but I *love* ice cream. And I admit, I used to eat ice cream way too often. Not as bad as my old twice a day meat and cheese habits, but ice cream every day in the summer was completely normal. I could swim and exercise all day, but 6 pack abs were not in the cards for my pre-CUSTOMIZE YOURSELF life. Eventually, I realized I'd be better off with less ice cream, so I thought, why not be creative? Why not make it a game? Make it a challenge to get the ice cream.

First, I would no longer fill up my freezer with ice cream. In the supermarket aisle, I would just... walk on by, don't stop, (again thanks Dionne, Burt and Hal). Works every time. But the notion of banning ice cream altogether seemed too radical. Nowadays, I go the extra mile. Back in 1921, RJR spent $8 million ($106 million in today's dollars) to launch the "I'd Walk a Mile for a Camel"

---

[131]Jimi Hendrix, "Purple Haze." *Are You Experienced*, Reprise Records, 1967.

advertising campaign for Camel cigarettes.[132]  I never saw anybody walk a mile for a cigarette.  I could never imagine a cigarette smoker walking a mile for anything.  Who knows if anybody ever walked a mile for a Camel?  But how about walking a mile for an ice cream cone?  I could do that.  In fact, I've done it many times.

My favorite ice cream is Kilwins.  Thank God, there isn't a Kilwins near me.  That would definitely make life more complicated.  There are a couple of Kilwins in the obscure regions of my state, but I ignore them.  I only go to one Kilwins.  The one in Delray Beach, Florida.  And since I live in New Jersey, it's a long walk.  About 1,210 miles if you take the less scenic route.  That's 2,420 miles round trip for 1 ice cream cone.  I won't say it's not worth it, but that's a long way to go for an ice cream cone.  If you *really* want to cut down on sugar though, that would be the way to do it.  Just walk 2,420 miles for each ice cream cone, and you'll be in great shape.  Try it.  Let me know how you make out.  I do it a little differently.  I fly to West Palm, take an Uber to Delray, get a room in a hotel that is about a half mile from Kilwins, walk the half mile to Kilwins, get an ice cream cone, then walk back to the hotel.  Mind you, I don't travel two thousand miles *just* for an ice cream cone.  I go to the beach, hit the gym, go out to dinner, stuff like that, but the highlight of the trip is definitely the Kilwins ice cream cone.

Try creating your own manic dessert challenge.  You can walk a half mile to the ice cream joint in your own town (and save a fortune on airfare, hotels, etc.), or do whatever seems like a fun challenge, or

---

[132] "Cigarettes," AD AGE, Sept. 15, 2003. https://adage.com/article/adage-encyclopedia/cigarettes/98574

passes as a positive, healthy endeavor to reduce the negative effects of your own slurping, Homer Simpson-esque activity.

## Coffee, Tea Or Ferrari?

Do you put sugar in your coffee or tea? One cup a day? Two? Three? More? Let's say you drink 2 cups a day. One teaspoon of sugar equals 4 grams. Two cups, 2 teaspoons, equals 8 grams. That's 56 grams per week, or 3.7 pounds a year. Use 2 teaspoons in your beverage, and you're up to 7.4 pounds a year. That's more than 1 of those 5 pound bales of sugar you almost get a hernia from lugging home from the supermarket. If you put more sugar in your coffee or tea, you'll need more bales of sugar, more hernias, and you'll never be able to afford that sports car.

You know you'd be way better off without all that extra sugar. What about a different sweetener? A low or no-calorie sugar-free replacement? According to an analysis of 37 studies published in the CANADIAN MEDICAL ASSOCIATION JOURNAL, using sweeteners like saccharin, aspartame and sucralose has been linked to weight gain, increases in waist circumference, and higher incidence of obesity, hypertension, metabolic syndrome, type 2 diabetes and cardiovascular events.[133] [134]

If you absolutely, positively must add some sweetener to your coffee or tea, try stevia. People in Paraguay and Brazil have used stevia leaves to sweeten food for centuries. After Japan banned artificial sweeteners more than 50 years ago, stevia was embraced as a safe substitute. It has been widely used there and other parts of Asia too. After hundreds of studies there and in the United States and Europe, stevia appears to be a much better choice than sugar.[135] It's use has risen tremendously in all sorts of food production globally.

When I decided to wean myself off adding sugar to my coffee, I tried stevia. While your market may only carry a few varieties of stevia, I would strongly suggest checking out at least a few health food stores, and trying out a whole bunch. Some taste awful, some taste good, and a few are just about as tasty and satisfying as sugar. Many of the most widely available brands are highly processed,

---

[133] Meghan Azad, lead author, "Nonnutritive sweeteners and cardiometabolic health: a systematic review and meta-analysis of randomized controlled trials and prospective cohort studies," CMAJ, July 17, 2017.
https://www.cmaj.ca/content/189/28/E929

[134] Marygrace Taylor, "8 Big Lies About Sugar We Should Unlearn," HEALTHLINE, Updated: Aug. 19, 2020.
https://www.healthline.com/health/food-nutrition/sugar-facts-scientific#10

[135] Hannah Nichols, "What is stevia?" MEDICAL NEWS TODAY, Jan. 4, 2018.
https://www.medicalnewstoday.com/articles/287251

contain additives and use genetically modified ingredients.[136] [137] Again, the best health food purveyors will carry ones that don't. Dosage can be a significant issue. Even some of the best liquid versions sold by reliable sources suggest 10 drops for your cup of joe when 1 or 2 drops will do just fine. After acclimating to 2 drops, it's easy to CUSTOMIZE YOURSELF down to 1 drop, (no party necessary, but an OK excuse to throw one).

And if you're on the hunt for food products without sugar, but crave sweetening, look for ingredient labels that have stevia alone, without other added sweeteners.

I discovered how to most comfortably and easily eliminate sweeteners from my morning coffee by accident. After gradually reducing my sugar fix to about a half teaspoon, then switching to stevia, and gradually reducing the stevia dosage, I got into the habit of carrying a packet of stevia with me when travelling. Some of the liquid versions taste much better, but not as convenient for pocket transportation. A fraction of a packet would provide a decent alternative. Then, one morning in Delray Beach, probably distracted by my fervent anticipation of an upcoming Kilwins visit, I not only found myself at the fabulous Seagate Hotel where they served the highly praised 'illy' coffee brand, but when I dug down for my pocket

---

[136] "Paraguayan plant stevia upends sugar market," REUTERS, Oct. 23, 2014. https://www.japantimes.co.jp/news/2014/10/23/world/science-health-world/paraguayan-plant-stevia-upends-sugar-market/#.XpR6qS-z1p8

[137] Natalie Digate Muth, MD, "The Truth About Stevia-The So-called 'Healthy' Alternative Sweetener," AMERICAN COUNCIL ON EXERCISE. https://www.acefitness.org/certifiednewsarticle/1644/the-truth-about-stevia-the-so-called-healthy-alternative-sweetener/

packet of stevia, it wasn't there. I had forgotten to bring my stash. No problem, I thought, a little sugar in my coffee, and it's no big deal. Here, I should mention that I had never tasted illy coffee. It's true that in my hedonistic youth, I would think nothing of dropping 45 or 50 bucks on a pound of Maui Kona or Jamaican Blue Mountain, which was absolutely fine with me until I figured out that I could actually go broke drinking coffee. So, as a mature adult, the idea of forking over 15 dollars for 8.8 ounce can of illy seemed to be a reckless proposition for home use. But there I was, at the fab Seagate, and they served illy coffee, and the grinning server swore it was the best coffee in the world. Yeah, sure kid, you ever drank Jamaican? Never mind. I got my cup of illy, reached for the sugar, and paused. If this coffee is so damn good, I wonder how it tastes *without* sugar. I poured in a few drops of milk to level the playing field, and took a sip. And wow, it was great. In one sip, I was off added sweeteners for the rest of my life. Oh, what a fool I had been. Thank you, illy. My point here is not to be a shill for illy or any other expensive coffee. No, it's just that a great coffee without sugar beats a mediocre coffee with sugar any day. Try a great coffee without sugar. If you make it a habit, your Ferrari purchase may be delayed, but your pancreas will thank you down the road.

## The Last Word On Sugar

The last word on sugar goes to Thomas L. Friedman, three-time Pulitzer Prize winning author, NEW YORK TIMES columnist, myth-buster, solution-seeker and problem-solver extraordinaire.

In his book, THANK YOU FOR BEING LATE: FINDING A JOB, RUNNING A COUNTRY, AND KEEPING YOUR HEAD IN AN AGE OF ACCELERATIONS,[138] Friedman argues for slashing all corporate taxes, income taxes, personal deductions and corporate subsidies, and replacing them with taxes on *sugar*, carbon, bullets and a small financial transaction tax.[139] His hypothetical "Mother Nature Party" advocates for entrepreneurism, pluralism and sustainability, traits that are easily observable in nature. "Climate will kill us, sugar will kill us, bullets will kill us, financial disruption will kill us."[140]

---

[138] Thomas L. Friedman, *Thank You for Being Late: An Optimist's Guide to Thriving in the Age of Accelerations.* New York: Farrar, Straus and Giroux, 2016.

[139] Thomas L. Friedman, "Up With Extremism," THE NEW YORK TIMES, Jan. 6, 2016. https://www.nytimes.com/2016/01/06/opinion/up-with-extremism.html

[140] William Morris, "Thomas Friedman: Society should mimic nature to survive," FINANCE & COMMERCE, Apr. 30, 2018. https://finance-commerce.com/2018/04/thomas-friedman-society-should-mimic-nature-to-thrive/

Sign me up for the Mother Nature Party.

## Can We Crystallize the Salt Situation?

You can live very well without sugar, but salt is necessary for good health.

What are the guidelines for the proper amount of daily sodium intake?

It depends on who you ask.

The American Heart Association recommends that healthy adults consume 1.5 grams (1,500 mg) a day, so does the Institute of Medicine. The World Health Organization suggests 2 grams a day. The USDA and US Department of Health and Human Services recommend limiting intake to less than 2.3 grams a day, equal to 1 teaspoon of salt.[141]  Americans consume an average of 3.4 grams of salt per day, 48% more than the USDA recommended amount.[142]  The

---

[141] Gavin Van De Walle, "How Much Sodium Should You Have per Day?" HEALTHLINE, Dec. 8, 2018. https://www.healthline.com/nutrition/sodium-per-day

[142] "You May Be Surprised by How Much Salt You're Eating," FDA Regulated Products, July 19, 2016. https://www.fda.gov/consumers/consumer-updates/you-may-be-surprised-how-much-salt-youre-eating

Heart Foundation in Australia recommends adults eat less than 5 grams of salt a day.[143]

So if you're hooked on salty foods, I guess you'll just have to move to Australia. Your blood pressure may not change, but Down Under you can chow down a crocodile, definitely a low-sodium reptile, only 51 mg of sodium per serving.[144]

While disagreement exists regarding what constitutes the ideal daily amount of sodium, it is widely accepted that excessive salt intake is a cause of high blood pressure. Not everyone responds to sodium in the same way. Several studies have indicated that not enough salt can worsen health more than consuming too much.[145] [146]

If you're an athlete and you sweat a lot, you need more salt. How much more salt? There is no proven formula for this. And keeping track of your salt intake is no easy chore either. Almost everything you buy that is processed or prepared has added salt. Bread, cold cuts, bacon, cheese, pasta and practically every dish coming out of a

---

[143] "Is salt bad for your heart?" HEART FOUNDATION. https://www.heartfoundation.org.au/healthy-eating/food-and-nutrition/salt/sodium-and-salt-converter

[144] "How many calories in Crocodile, Tail Fillet, raw," CALORIEKING. https://www.calorieking.com/au/en/foods/f/calories-in-game-crocodile-tail-fillet-raw/PyU5vTLXRsOpL_tVbZsFpA

[145] Gavin Van De Walle, "How Much Sodium Should You Have per Day?" HEALTHLINE, Dec. 8, 2018. https://www.healthline.com/nutrition/sodium-per-day

[146] Andrew Mente, lead author, "Associations of urinary sodium excretion with cardiovascular events in individuals with and without hypertension: a pooled analysis of data from four studies," LANCET, July 30, 2016; 388(10043): 465-75. https://www.ncbi.nlm.nih.gov/pubmed/27216139

restaurant kitchen has extra salt. One tablespoon of soy sauce contains 1 gram of sodium. You can exceed your daily limit with a short sit at the sushi bar. A stack of a chocolate chip pancakes can clock in at 2 grams of salt. A bagel is in the range of 460-600 mg of salt. When you see "reduced sodium" on a label, according to FDA rules, it means that a food has only 25% less sodium than the original product; so for a food product that has 1 gram of salt, the "reduced sodium" version would have 750 mg. Many foods naturally contain salt including fruits, vegetables, dairy products, meat and shellfish. And some common foods have unusually high sodium content. A lowly cup of low-fat cottage cheese boasts 1 gram of sodium.[147] It all adds up.

The CDC has concluded that sodium intake from processed and restaurant foods contributes to high rates of high blood pressure, heart attack and stroke; and sodium reduction continues to be an effective and safe way to lower blood pressure.[148]

Different people retain salt differently. It may be argued that if you do not have high blood pressure, then your daily salt intake is probably not too high. I'll go with the CDC, and accept that most people would benefit by reducing their salt intake, but there seems to be no perfect blueprint for every individual. Your doctor can best advise you.

---

[147] Jessica Girdwain, "13 Foods That Are Saltier Than You Realize," HEALTH, Oct. 31, 2014. https://www.health.com/nutrition/13-foods-that-are-saltier-than-you-realize?

[148] "How does salt affect blood pressure?" Heart Disease, Sodium. Centers for Disease Control and Prevention, cdc.gov, https://www.cdc.gov/heartdisease/sodium.htm

# WARNING: READ THE LABEL OR DIE!

Or at least you'll die sooner than if you don't read labels. I know, I can't prove it, but I believe it's true. If you don't read labels, you will consume astronomical quantities of added sodium and sugars, a dizzying array of chemicals, additives, thickening agents, extracts, trans fats, flavor enhancers, dyes, artificial sweeteners, including a whole bunch of stuff that has not been deemed dangerous by the FDA for human consumption, but given the choice, most people would find about as appetizing as roadkill. Stuff like calcium sulfate, which is quite simply, plaster, also know as gypsum. A fine building material, calcium sulfate is also commonly added to tofu products, breakfast cereals, bakery products, pastas, hot dogs, batters, diet products and many beverages including alcoholic beverages, and energy/sports drinks.[149]

Caveat emptor. Let the buyer beware. And let's make it even simpler. You don't have to read the *whole* label, just the ingredients. In fact, you'd probably be better off ignoring everything on the label except the ingredients. Food product labels commonly make

---

[149] Jessica Bruso, 'What Foods Contain Calcium Sulfate?" LIVESTRONG.COM, https://www.livestrong.com/article/254242-what-foods-contain-calcium-sulfate/

excessive claims that are often false or misleading. 'Natural' may hardly be natural at all, it's merely an implication that some natural source is involved or included. 'No added sugar' does not mean a product is not high in sugar, it may contain unhealthy sugar substitutes. 'Low-calorie' products need to have one-third less calories than the brand's original product, which could still be a lot of calories in comparison to other brands' offerings. 'Low-fat' may be high-calorie with added sugar. 'Fortified' may indicate a vitamin or mineral has been added, but that does not necessarily make it a healthy product. 'Gluten-free' foods can be highly processed with high amounts of starch, sugar, salt and unhealthy fats. 'Zero trans fat' only signifies that a *serving* has under .5 grams of trans fat; if the servings are tiny, that number can get multiplied. If a serving size is one-quarter of a cookie with seemingly low amounts of sugar and calories, just eat two cookies, and those low amounts are now multiplied *eight*-fold. 'Fruit-flavored' may only contain chemicals that taste like fruit; actual fruit is not required.[150]

The food industries in the United States and most of the rest of the world have gone berserk adding excessive, unnecessary amounts of sugar and salt to everything imaginable. And they have fought to make label ingredients as confusing as possible. Food manufacturers have developed and deployed a creative crapload of monikers for sugar. You'll see beet sugar, brown sugar, cane sugar, invert sugar, organic raw sugar, coconut sugar, confectioner's sugar, evaporated

---

[150] Adda Bjarnadottir, "How to Read Food Labels Without Being Tricked" HEALTHLINE, Updated: Aug. 19, 2020.
https://www.healthline.com/nutrition/how-to-read-food-labels

cane juice, high-fructose corn syrup, malt syrup, maple syrup, oat syrup, rice syrup, rice bran syrup, brown rice syrup, honey, agave nectar, barley malt, molasses, dextrose, fructose, lactose, maltose, glucose, sucrose, corn sweetener, and maltodextrin (which is a triple whammy sweetener/thickener/preservative that can change your gut bacteria composition,  suppress the growth of probiotics in your digestive system, and can increase the growth of bacteria such as E. coli which is associated with autoimmune disorders like Crohn's disease).[151] [152]   And the list goes on, and on, and on.

Do you buy almond milk?   See if you can find a variety *without* added sugar.  The vast majority have added sugars.  Some have a lot of added sugar.  Is it really necessary to add sugar to almond milk, coconut milk, soy milk or any plant-based milk?

What about cereal?  Try to find a box of cornflakes without added salt or sugar.  Impossible.  Try to find a box of any kind of cereal anywhere in America without added salt or sugar.  Nearly impossible. I visited one of the biggest supermarkets in New Jersey housing an extensive "Natural Foods" section with a long aisle of shelves packed with "natural" cereals.  I tried to find one single box of cereal that had less than 6% sugar.  I could not find one.  Most were much higher than 6%, plenty had over 10% sugar content.   Pretty depressing.

---

[151] Anna Shaefer, "Is Maltodextrin bad for Me?", HEALTHLINE, Sept. 12, 2018. https://www.healthline.com/health/food-nutrition/is-maltodextrin-bad-for-me

[152] Kourtney Nickerson, Christine McDonald, "Crohn's Disease-Associated Adherent-Invasive *Escherichia coli* Adhesion Is Enhanced by Exposure to the Ubiquitous Dietary Polysaccharide Maltodextrin," PLOS ONE, Dec. 12, 2012. https://journals.plos.org/plosone/article?id=10.1371/journal.pone.0052132

Surprisingly, I found many boxes of cereal in the "regular" cereal aisle that had *less* sugar than the much more expensive ones in the "natural" section. What's going on here? Why are these "natural" food producers adding so much cheap sugar to their expensive products? Maybe they should change the name of the "Natural Foods" section to the "Sugar Foods" section.

How about a visit to the canned goods section?

No soup for you!

Well, no soup for me anyway. You can still have soup, but you may pause after reading the ingredients. Following my trip down the "natural" cereal/sugar aisle, I visited the lengthy soup aisle. I could not find a single can that had less 600 mg of salt. And the one that had 600 mg, proudly proclaimed on the front of the can that is was "low sodium." Not a single soup maker had the courage to put a little or no salt in their product. They must be convinced that we could not possibly want their soup without a load of salt. I can't even imagine how much salt is contained in the supermarket-made, plastic containers of soup in the prepared foods section. Maybe I should have stuck my own label on their containers, "If you knew how much salt was in this, you wouldn't buy it." Homemade soup, on the other hand, is a godsend. You don't have to load it with salt, and you can benefit from all the nutrients that are not as obtainable from raw vegetables. Cooking tomatoes increases the bioavailability of the antioxidant lycopene by a factor of *five*. The beta-carotene in cooked carrots is also more available for the body to assimilate. And, cooking spinach will increase iron and calcium absorption.[153]

Now that we're having fun reading labels, see if you can find Polysorbate 80, monosodium glutamate (MSG), butylated hydroxy anisole (BHA), butylated hydroxytoluene (BHT), sodium nitrate, sodium nitrite, propyl gallate, sodium benzoate, benzoic acid, potassium bromate, or some other polysyllabic imprint on a label that doesn't make your mouth water. While not banned by the FDA, these additives have generated a myriad controversies among many detractors. Add to the above an endless rainbow of food colorings, some derived from natural substances, and some derived from petroleum. Red #3, red #40, yellow #5 and yellow #6 have received special attention in many studies for demonstrating chromosomal damage, tumors and lymphomas.[154]

If you make it as far as the frozen foods aisle, you may find ingredient labels even more vexing with even more syllables. And while you're reading them, your fingers will freeze quite possibly along with your brain. A typical 2,000 calorie frozen pizza can clock in at 5 grams of sodium, along with its share of unpronounceable extras. There is an abundance of conflicting data on the effects of a diet relying on frozen foods. Personally, I am quite happy to have abandoned the frozen foods section a long time ago. When I was an

---

[153] Christopher Wanjek, "Reality Check: 5 Risks of Raw Vegan Diet," LIVE SCIENCE, Jan. 15, 2013. https://www.livescience.com/26278-risks-raw-vegan-diet.html

[154] Cat Perry, "The 9 Scariest Food Additives You're Eating Right Now," MEN'S JOURNAL.COM, https://www.mensjournal.com/food-drink/9-scariest-food-additives-youre-eating-right-now/

overscheduled, nutritionally-challenged student, I often grabbed cheap frozen entrees to fill my gut. At an early stage of improving my diet, I quit the TV dinners and immediately noticed that I felt much better in general, more energetic, clearheaded, with better focus and concentration. I strongly advocate skipping frozen foods altogether.

For those of you who are not in the habit of reading labels, and those who may think that it's some sort of imposition on your precious time, once again, you simply begin your journey with the first step. Spend an extra 2 minutes in the market reading 2 labels per visit. Before you know it, you'll be an expert label-reader. You may get so good at it, you'll run out of labels to read. Remember, you only have to read a label *once* in your life. Subsequent perusals are optional. If you see excessive amounts of salt or sugar, chemicals, preservatives, dyes, gums, artificial anything, or other ingredients that you don't want, can't recognize, or have way too many syllables, put it back on the shelf. You're done with it. You've eliminated an undesirable concoction from your life. That's a good thing. Congratulations!

You may even want to adopt my label-gazing hypothesis, which is a rough cause and effect ratio of every minute you spend reading a label will add 1 day to your life, or something like that. Maybe it'll only add 5 minutes, you can decide for yourself. At least, you'll be more informed.[155]

---

[155] May also be considered Meshuga Theory #2. No study to quote here, but label-gazing is more instructive than navel-gazing.

# CALL TO ACTION!

It doesn't take a lot of label-reading to figure out that way too many food manufacturers will continue to add staggering amounts of sodium and sugar to their products as long as they can make a profit selling them. Just about any politician who may act like they want to do something about this unhealthy state of affairs will get a visit from one or many lobbyists with a variety of arguments and inducements to garner support. Or, said politician may soon be running against an opponent who was more receptive to said visiting lobbyist(s). Or, soda-guzzling fanatics and their defenders like Jon Stewart will storm the capitol steps and cause unhealthy outcomes. (I'm not blaming Jon Stewart for all the damage caused by sugary drinks. It's just that anyone with a microphone can be either be part of the problem or part of the solution. Also, I miss his inspired lunacy and righteous indignation on THE DAILY SHOW).

What can be done about this?

Make some noise!

If enough people complain, boycott and demand no salt and no sugar alternatives, the food industry will adapt. They want your business. Tell the food manufacturers what *you* want. They spend time, effort and money to get positive reviews all over social media. They may even take action after seeing an avalanche of negative reviews.  Tell your supermarket managers.  Tell the rack jobbers you see in the market packing the shelves with the stuff you don't want. Some of them will listen and take action.

Just imagine if you could buy everything you want salt-free and sugar-free, and then go home and have the freedom to decide if you want to add a sprinkle of salt or sugar, or not.  Season to taste.  Season to health.  Customize your food!

Meanwhile, spend as much of your grocery shopping time as possible on the perimeters of the supermarket.

Buy food, not food products.

Buy food made by nature, not factory chemists.

# The Plethora Of Plates, Pyramids And Percentages

For over 100 years, the U.S. Department of Agriculture (USDA) has published a long line of food guides, charts, wheels, pyramids and plates divided into food groups associated with expanding and contracting amounts and percentages, redefined at irregular intervals according to the compromises and conclusions made by the USDA and the dairy, meat, grain and other food lobbyists, and those politicians the lobbyists help elect. It's sort of like gerrymandering, but with food instead of voters. With gerrymandering, the politicians elect the voters. With food guidelines, the government elects the food. At various times, ketchup and tomato paste were deemed vegetables for school lunch programs.[156]

The most recent USDA derivation, called ChooseMyPlate, is connected to an array of online tools declaring early on that, "Any fruit or 100% fruit juice counts as a part of the Fruit Group," and, "Any vegetable or 100% vegetable juice counts as a member of the Vegetable Group."[157] They recommend that meals should have about

---

[156] Marion Nestle, "Ketchup Is a Vegetable? Again?" THE ATLANTIC, Nov. 16, 2011. https://www.theatlantic.com/health/archive/2011/11/ketchup-is-a-vegetable-again/248538/

[157] "ChooseMyPlate," USDA, https://www.choosemyplate.gov/

30% vegetables, 20% fruit and 30% grains.[158]  Most contemporary grain warriors are offended by this high percentage of grains, and advocate for more fruits and vegetables. You can follow USDA guidelines into a rabbit hole of definitions, declarations, combinations and recommendations, some very sensible, and some not.  It all seems to exist to somehow justify present and future behaviors and practices favored by institutions who may need to cover their asses.  I imagine that USDA scientists, if left to their own devices, without outside influence and interference, could build a  better mouse trap, but as it stands, it looks like something that works better for the food industry than the average citizen.

---

[158] "The Original Renewable Energy Source," Federal Occupational Health (FOH), PSC, U.S Department of Health and Human Services (HHS). https://foh.psc.gov/calendar/nutrition.html

## Some Of My Best Friends Are Plants

I definitely get along better with plants than with humans. I love plants. People, eh? While humans are busy gobbling and destroying oxygen and producing carbon dioxide, plants absorb carbon dioxide and produce oxygen as a waste product. Plants don't talk back. They don't take out college loans. They don't need car insurance, health insurance, Air Jordans, iPhones or braces. You don't have to bail them out of jail. They ask so little (just add water), and they give so much, merely, Life as we know it. Plants provide fantastic nourishment. Without plants, we lowly humans could not survive.

According to the CDC, about 90% of Americans don't eat enough fruits and vegetables.[159] And when you consider that many of the newest wave of nutrition advocates recommend eating in the range of 70-80% plant-based (some even higher), then over 90% of Americans are deficient in this vital regard.

---

[159] Seung Hee lee-Kwan, Ph.D., lead author, "Disparities in State-Specific Adult Fruit and Vegetable Consumption-United States,2015," CDC Morbidity and Mortality Weekly Report, Nov. 17, 2017.
https://www.cdc.gov/mmwr/volumes/66/wr/mm6645a1.htm?s_cid=mm6645a1_w&utm_source=STAT+Newsletters&utm_campaign=f26644060f-MR&utm_medium=email&utm_term=0_8cab1d7961-f26644060f-150444909

Increasing plant-based intake while at the same time reducing or avoiding sugar and flour is a simple, sensible, general plan of attack to improve health and well-being.

Eating fruits and vegetables in season also has many benefits. Freshness, flavor and nutrition can be maximized by purchasing from local growers soon after harvest. Storing foods for long periods often causes significant loses of vitamin content and antioxidants.[160] Buying produce from distant locales necessitates additional transportation costs, and creates more global warming emissions.

---

[160] Divya Ramaswamy, "7 Reasons Why Should You Eat Seasonal Fruits And Vegetables," INTERNATIONAL BUSINESS TIMES, Oct. 17, 2019. https://www.ibtimes.com/7-reasons-why-should-you-eat-seasonal-fruits-vegetables-2848027

## You Say Potato


If you've spent any time with all the media-savvy health gurus and self-appointed pundits promoting their programs, books, DVD's, supplements, recipes, declarations, holy advice, rules and warnings, your head is already spinning. When you drill down into their proclamations about which fruits and vegetables are good for you, and which ones are bad for you, the conflicts and contradictions cause more confusion, and shred credibility. I have reached a point where I know I should stop paying attention to the drone of health-hawkers, but it's hard to look away. It's like watching plant-based crash scene, but instead of rubbernecking delays caused by planes, trains and automobiles, it's potatoes, tomatoes and kidney beans.

You can now find a bunch of the biggest-selling nutrition and health book authors bashing potatoes, telling their readers not to eat them, while others say the opposite.

Potatoes are packed with nutrients and antioxidants, may improve digestive health, are gluten-free, cheap, and they fill you up.[161] Fried potatoes have issues, (see: 'French Fries and Married Guys'), but a

---

[161] Ryan Raman, "7 Health and Nutrition Benefits of Potatoes," HEALTHLINE, Mar. 14, 2018. https://www.healthline.com/nutrition/benefits-of-potatoes#section6

simple baked potato is great. Load it up with piles of butter, cheese and sour cream, not so great. Many studies have participants consuming baked, mashed *and* fried potatoes. Some studies suggest that diabetics could benefit from potato-related blood sugar control.[162] [163] Others claim potatoes' high glycemic index (GI) makes it a food to avoid.[164] And The American Journal of Clinical Nutrition found that, "…there is substantial variability in individual responses to GI value determination, demonstrating that it is unlikely to be a good approach to guiding food choices."[165]

So how do we approach the above-ground potato? The stuffed potato sack of associations, accusations and varied data is confusing. One might say, different potato strokes for different potato folks. I say, baked or boiled, and once in a while, mashed (easy on the butter/milk/salt).

Over in the data patch of tomato studies, many extoll the virtues of tomatoes. This it's-a-fruit, no, it's-a-vegetable, OK, it's a fruit, but

---

[162] Ibid.

[163] Chia-Hung Lin, lead author, "Assessment of Blood Glucose Regulation and Safety of Resistant Starch Formula-Based Diet in Healthy Normal and Subjects With Type 2 Diabetes," MEDICINE, Aug. 21, 2015. https://www.ncbi.nlm.nih.gov/pmc/articles/PMC4616456/

[164] Jessie Szalay, "Potatoes: Health Benefits, Risks & Nutrition Facts," LIVE SCIENCE, Oct. 24, 2017. https://www.livescience.com/45838-potato-nutrition.html

[165] Nirupa Matthan, lead author, "Estimating the reliability of glycemic index values and potential sources of methodological and biological variability," THE AMERICA JOURNAL OF CLINICAL NUTRITION, Vol. 104, Issue 4, Oct. 2016, pp. 1004-1013. https://academic.oup.com/ajcn/article/104/4/1004/4557132

everyone thinks it's a vegetable and treats it like a vegetable, but does-it-really-matter popular orb is an excellent source of lycopene, vitamin C, potassium, folate, vitamin K, beta-carotene and fiber. Tomatoes have been linked with heart health, cancer prevention and skin health. But have you ever wondered why commercially grown tomatoes taste like Styrofoam? It's because they're harvested and transported while still green. Then to make them red before selling, food companies spray them with artificial ethylene gas. Yum! This inhibits the development of natural flavor, and can make brilliant red tomatoes that look beautiful but taste ugly. Again, if at all possible, it's best to buy locally, and ripen naturally.[166]

Among the anti-tomato group, fit and famous, plant-based consumers, Tom Brady and Gisele Bundchen consume 80% vegetables, but won't eat tomatoes. Brady believes his tomato-free diet will enable him to remain a top quarterback deep into his forties.[167] And, various claims have been made that eating tomatoes can cause all sorts of problems including kidney stones, joint pain, acid reflux and histamine-related allergic reactions.[168]

---

[166] Adda Bjarnadottir, "Tomatoes 101: Nutrition Facts and Health Benefits," HEALTHLINE, Mar. 25, 2019.
https://www.healthline.com/nutrition/foods/tomatoes

[167] Julia Belluz, "Tom Brady's diet book makes some strange claims about body chemistry," VOX, Updated: Feb. 1, 2019.
https://www.vox.com/2019/1/30/18203676/tom-brady-diet-book-water

[168] Leian Naduma, "7 Shocking Side Effects of Eating Tomatoes Excessively," MEDICAL DAILY, May 16, 2019. https://www.medicaldaily.com/adverse-effects-eating-excess-tomatoes-434837

Why is it that potatoes and tomatoes continue to arouse bounties of controversies and love/hate reactions?

Is it because potato and tomato rhyme?

Or maybe we should blame Fred Astaire and Ginger Rogers,

*You like potato and I like potahto*
*You like tomato and I like tomahto*
*Potato, potahto, tomato, tomahto!*
*Let's call the whole thing off![169]*

I know, before your time. Mine too. But if you are unable to consume a tomato without questioning its efficacy or your chances of playing in the NFL, see if you can figure out whether Fred Astaire could dance better than Tom Brady can throw a football. (Answer in footnote).[170]

As with the often maligned potato, the tomato has its detractors, but personally, no one could talk me out of eating tomatoes (well, maybe Gisele Bundchen). A real Jersey tomato is the stuff of legend, (although I once had a Florida heirloom tomato so suspiciously delicious that I wonder if it may have been snuck in from New Jersey). From the 1930s to the 1970s the 'Rutgers' and the 'Ramapo' tomato

---

[169] George Gershwin and Ira Gershwin. "Let's Call the Whole Thing Off." *Shall We Dance*, RKO Radio Pictures, 1937.

[170] The answer is complicated. You have to first determine whether Brady would be so good if he wasn't married to Gisele Bundchen. Then, you have to consider that most experts claim Fred Astaire was the greatest dancer in the history of movies. And, if you accept that, you have to explain how Ginger Rogers could dance as well as Fred Astaire, but backwards, in heels.

varieties made New Jersey famous. Then Bruce Springsteen came along, and Jersey tomatoes' glory days were, like it goes in the song,

*Glory days*
*Well they'll pass you by, glory days*
*In the wink of a young girl's eye, glory days*
*Glory days*[171]

'Rutgers' and 'Ramapo' were developed at the Rutgers New Jersey Agricultural Experiment Station.[172] If you are a serious tomato grower or merely an aficionado, you can follow their research and breeding efforts here: http://forms.feedblitz.com/33w

Back underground, in the moist world of tubers, the journey burrows on. As I have been gradually reducing my grain/flour/gluten intakes, and seeking to embrace better alternatives, I have rediscovered the wonders of the fabulous sweet potato. Sweet potatoes are an excellent source of fiber, potassium, vitamin C and a highly absorbable variety of beta carotene. More intensely orange sweet potatoes have a higher beta carotene content and are credited

---

[171] Bruce Springsteen, "Glory Days." *Born in the U.S.A.,* Columbia Records, 1984.

[172] "Rutgers NJAES: All-Star Varieties, Tomatoes," Rutgers New Jersey Agricultural Experiment Station. https://breeding.rutgers.edu/tomatoes/

with increasing blood levels of vitamin A.[173] [174]  They are heralded by most potato dissenters mainly because sweet potatoes have a lower glycemic index (GI) than potatoes.  A perfectly baked sweet potato requires little effort and no talent.  It's delicious all by itself, and needs no butter or cheese or anything.

Bear in mind, most root vegetables are also starches, so don't overdo them.  Too many carbs in one meal can spike blood sugar.  And if you consume more carbohydrates than your body needs, they will be stored as fat, leading to weight gain.[175]

A variety of root vegetables is desirable.  But once again, to best CUSTOMIZE YOURSELF, consider what you like, and pay attention to what likes you.  I really, really don't like beets and radishes.  Garlic and onions really don't like me.  Even a bite is like a gut punch.  Ginger, I can handle a little.  Turmeric certainly has its boosters.  Turmeric contains the chemical curcumin.  This and other chemicals in turmeric have been linked with an incredible array of health claims including possibly reducing hay fever symptoms and joint pain, lowering triglycerides, promoting better liver function, treating depression, PMS and osteoarthritis, improving mental

---

[173] Adda Bjarnadottir, "Sweet Potatoes 101: Nutrition Facts and Health Benefits," HEALTHLINE, May 13, 2019.
https://www.healthline.com/nutrition/foods/sweet-potatoes

[174] F Jalal, lead author, "Serum retinol concentrations in children are affected by food sources of beta-carotene, fat intake, and anthelmintic drug treatment," THE AMERICAN JOURNAL OF CLINICAL NUTRITION, 1998 Sep;68(3):623-9.  https://www.ncbi.nlm.nih.gov/pubmed/9734739

[175] "The pros and cons of root vegetables," HARVARD HEALTH LETTER, Aug. 2018.  https://www.health.harvard.edu/staying-healthy/the-pros-and-cons-of-root-vegetables

function in older adults, lowering risks of digestive disorders, diabetes and some cancers, and a whole bunch more.[176] To maximize turmeric's benefits, adding black pepper has been shown to increase absorption in your gut.[177] It's no secret that the purveyors of turmeric are giddy with their praise, many claiming that it is the most effective nutritional supplement on earth.

However, in the midst of the COVID-19 pandemic, the French Agency for Food, Environmental and Occupational Health and Safety (ANSES) cited several plants including turmeric (and echinacea and liquorice) with anti-inflammatory properties as being, "…capable of disturbing the body's natural defenses which are useful in fighting infections and, in particular, against COVID-19." ANSES recommended that people with a preventative aim in mind suspend consumption of food supplements containing these plants as soon as the first symptoms of COVID-19 appear.[178]

More study awaits, and the saga of turmeric shall continue. Perhaps one day, Netflix will produce a hit series on turmeric (if they can find the right actor who looks good in orange powder).

---

[176] "Turmeric," WebMD,
https://www.webmd.com/vitamins/ai/ingredientmono-662/turmeric

[177] Guido Shoba, lead author, "Influence of piperine on the pharmacokinetics of curcumin in animals and human volunteers," Department of Pharmacology, St. John's Medical College, Bangalore, India, Oct. 18, 1997.
https://pdfs.semanticscholar.org/e47f/5da58f0276bddd54b9575938e6cbad
65a31d.pdf?_ga=2.133009229.21864851.1607893531-
1758067182.1607893531

[178] Will Chu, "ANSES warns of turmeric-based supplements' effect on immune response," NUTRAingredients.com, Updated: Apr. 20, 2020.
https://www.nutraingredients.com/Article/2020/04/20/ANSES-warns-of-
turmeric-supplement-effect-on-immune-response#

My biggest plug for a root vegetable goes to carrots. Super nutritious, high in beta-carotene, vitamins A and K, I am hooked on carrots. Carrots were my entry vegetable. From carrots, I moved on to spinach, string beans and asparagus. While I give my mother credit for presenting and promoting a wide array of nourishing vegetables in my formative years, she was not terribly successful at convincing me of their vital necessity. Anytime she offered me a carrot, I sort of leaned to the side, trying to see behind her, into the pantry, where a box of Ring Dings might be hidden on a high shelf. I would only accept the carrot out of sheer hunger and desperation. This pathetic ritual continued until the day my innocent world was shattered by a Warner Bros. cartoon. It starred Bugs Bunny. Wow! Bugs was so cool. And he wielded a carrot better than Humphrey Bogart could brandish a cigarette. "Ehh, what's up doc?" was not only one of the greatest lines in cinema, Bugs owned it. No one else could have it, use it, steal it, exploit it, it was all Bugs. Elmer Fudd could stick a shotgun in his face, ready to blow his brains out, and Bugs would calmly take a bite of his carrot, pause for a few chomps, smile, and disarm with a nonchalant, "Ehh, what's up doc?" Changed my outlook on life. And death. And carrots. And vegetables altogether.

# Do You Choose Your Friends Or Do They Choose You?

*The sport I originally chose was baseball.*
*But it didn't choose me back.*
*And that, as Robert Frost would say,*
*has made all the difference.*
*-Kareem Abdul-Jabbar* [179]

My guess is that most people think they choose their friends, but will admit that they don't always make the best choices. I remember when one of my friends told me, "You can pick your friends, and you can pick your nose, but you can't pick your friend's nose." I thought that was brilliant until it became apparent that I wasn't always able to pick my friends, therefore it did not follow that, I could *not* pick my nose, or that I *could* pick my friend's nose. Now, just for fun, let's reconsider the 'What Likes You?' chapter, and assume that some people just don't like you, and some foods don't like you either.

Many cruciferous vegetables, most notably broccoli and cauliflower, have been branded '"superfoods," which is not an actual food group, but really an overused marketing term for foods with

---

[179] NBA Hall of Famer Kareem Abdul-Jabbar, "Two Summer Binges for Sports-Starved Fans," *The Hollywood Reporter*, July 8, 2020, p. 41.

dense nutritional value. And make no mistake, broccoli and cauliflower deserve the attention. Both are rich in fiber, vitamins A, C and K, folate, and an assortment of carotenoids like beta-carotene, lutein and zeaxanthin, and universally credited with antioxidant benefits. But they can be challenging to digest, and cause gas. Cruciferous vegetables have sulfur-containing chemicals called glucosinolates which break down in the intestines to form compounds like hydrogen sulfide which add the smell of sulfur to passing gas. Cruciferous vegetables also contain raffinose, a sugar that humans don't have the enzyme to digest. Raffinose enters the large intestine undigested, and often results in gas and bloating.[180]

The severity of these reactions varies among individuals. You have to weigh the benefits, and judge for yourself. I actually like broccoli and cauliflower, and would eat them regularly, except neither of them likes me. Since I prefer to live without stomach pain and excessive farting, I avoid them. None of the products that claim to reduce gas caused by cruciferous vegetables work very well, certainly not for me. So, adios broccoli and cauliflower. If broccoli or cauliflower may be objectionable to you, with hardly any detective work, you can find other "superfoods," even within the highly touted cruciferous vegetable group, that are fine substitutes. I discovered that my new friends,

kale and arugula treated me a lot better, so we bonded, and plan dinner together whenever we can.

---

[180] Jessica Cording, "Want To Avoid Gas & Bloating At Holiday Parties? Don't Eat This Healthy Food," MINDBODYGREEN.
https://www.mindbodygreen.com/articles/how-cruciferous-vegetables-can-cause-gas-and-bloating

Similar digestive challenges commonly arise with beans and legumes. Chickpeas, lentils, black beans, fava beans, kidney beans, lima beans, navy beans, pinto beans, soybeans, peas and peanuts contain considerable quantities of fiber, protein, folate, thiamine, calcium, iron, manganese, magnesium, zinc, copper and potassium, while in many individuals frequently trigger bloating and flatulence.[181] For the fart-adverse, testing your digestive reactions with small amounts is a good approach. You'll probably discover some friendly beans and legumes along with the unfriendly ones. My own gut checks have resulted in warm relations with lentils, chickpeas and peanuts while taking it very easy with most of the dry beans. And I remain forever suspicious of fava beans since Hannibal Lecter's creepy endorsement.[182]

The point here is that no one has to suffer unnecessarily because they have been lectured about why they should eat a particular food. You choose. Try new stuff. Listen to your gut. Feel the burn. Smell the room. Figure it out. CUSTOMIZE YOURSELF.

---

[181] "Meat or beans: What will you have? Part II: Beans," HARVARD MEN'S HEALTH WATCH, Mar. 2011. https://www.health.harvard.edu/staying-healthy/meat-or-beans-what-will-you-have-part-ll-beans

[182] "I ate his liver with fava beans and chianti." Hannibal Lecter (Anthony Hopkins) to Clarice Starling (Jodie Foster) in *The Silence of the Lambs,* Orion Pictures, 1991.

# Green Is Good

'Green Is Good' should have been the most famous line in WALL STREET.

Actually, Michael Douglas said, "*Greed*, for lack of a better word, is good."[183] I think *Green* is the better word. 'The Big Salad' only hinted at the tremendous variety of green vegetables that you should be trying out on your gut. My introduction to super-fibrous greens occurred naturally in the City of Angels, right after I wiped out my student loan-fortified bank account paying tuition at the University of Southern California. I visited the produce aisle in the local market, and could not help noticing that it looked a whole lot different than the ones in New Jersey. It was stacked with bargain-priced collard greens, mustard greens, turnip greens, and all sorts of dense green stuff I hadn't see in the 'burbs of Jersey. They're great in salads, delivering maximum nutrition raw, although breaking down a load of raw collard greens is a challenge for anyone's gut. Mustard greens go down easier. Nowadays, kale, spinach, romaine lettuce, swiss chard, endive, bok choy and arugula have become widely available and very popular. Loaded with vitamins, especially high in vitamins

---

[183] Gordon Gecko (Michael Douglas) in *Wall Street,* Twentieth Century Fox, 1987.

A, C and K, minerals, antioxidants and fiber, all of these leafy greens should be sampled. No formal introductions necessary. Make some friends!

And if you really want to max out your vitamin intake, enter the world of microgreens. Considered baby plants, microgreens are grown in soil, usually harvested 2 or 3 weeks after germination, reaching heights of 1 to 3 inches, and can be grown outdoors, in greenhouses or even on a window sill. Seed producers have developed a wide array of plant and cereal seeds for purchase. Introduced mostly as a garnish in trendy California restaurants in the 1980s, microgreens have gained widespread acceptance as significant food sources to enhance salads, sandwiches and entrees. They boast a wide variety of flavors, from neutral to spicy, sour and bitter.[184] Several studies have found that almost all of the microgreens have much higher concentrations of nutrients than the mature leaves of the same plant.[185] [186]

---

[184] Alina Petre, "Microgreens: All You Ever Wanted to Know," HEALTHLINE, Mar. 6, 2018. https://www.healthline.com/nutrition/microgreens#what-are-they

[185] Eliza Barclay, "Introducing Microgreens: Younger, And Maybe More Nutritious Vegetables," NPR, Aug. 30, 2012. https://www.npr.org/sections/thesalt/2012/08/29/160274163/introducing-microgreens-younger-and-maybe-more-nutritious-vegetables

[186] Zhenlei Xeao, lead author, "Assessment of Vitamin and Carotenoid Concentrations of Emerging Food Products: Edible Microgreens," JOURNAL OF AGRICULTURAL AND FOOD CHEMISTRY, July 18, 2012. http://www.sweetcitymicros.com/uploads/1/1/7/0/117059123/nutrient_levels.pdf

## Grow Your Own

If you have any kind of access to a patch of soil, you should be growing your own vegetables and fruits. It's as local as you can get, and the taste, nutrition and satisfaction of a job well done are among the greatest rewards life can offer.

Equally vital is to populate your indoor life with plants. House plants make your interior confines come alive physically, mentally and aesthetically. Plants absorb carbon dioxide and release oxygen indoors too. They add moisture, increasing humidity indoors, especially welcome during drier months and in closed-window environments, which is also helpful in reducing dry skin, colds, sore throats and dry coughs.[187]

A study at Texas A&M University concluded that being around plants increases memory retention and concentration at home and in the workplace. "Work performed under the natural influence of ornamental plants is normally of higher quality and completed with a

---

[187] Melissa Breyer, "5 Health Benefits of Houseplants," TREEHUGGER, Updated: Nov. 23, 2020. https://www.treehugger.com/health/5-health-benefits-houseplants.html

much higher accuracy rate than work done in environments devoid of nature."[188]

Plants can boost healing too. A study conducted at Kansas State University found that plants in hospital rooms enhanced health outcomes of patients recovering from surgery.[189] Just think about all the things you'll be recovering from for the rest of your life, and the ready-to-nurture ability of your plants to care for you!

NASA research has shown that indoor plant leaves can remove low levels of toxic chemicals like formaldehyde (which unfortunately is still widely used in adhesives, building products, rugs, drapes, fabrics, furniture, cabinets, pressed-wood products, flooring, cosmetics, detergents and many other objects commonly found everyone's homes).[190] Concluding that astronauts need fresh fruits and vegetables in space as well as on earth, NASA is now growing space station plants with their Vegetable Production System known as Veggie. NASA has documented the nutritional benefits as well as "enhancing happiness and well-being on the orbiting laboratory." They have successfully grown a variety of lettuces, Chinese cabbage,

---

[188] "Health and well-being benefits of plants," Ellison Chair in International Floriculture, Texas A&M Agrilife Extension.
https://ellisonchair.tamu.edu/health-and-well-being-benefits-of-plants/#.VN4ge-ddVfA

[189] Seong-Hyun Park, Richard Mattson, "Ornamental indoor plants in hospital rooms enhanced health outcomes of patients recovering from surgery," JOURNAL OF ALTERNATIVE AND COMPLEMENTARY MEDICINE, Sept. 15, 2009, 15(9), pp. 975-980.
https://www.ncbi.nlm.nih.gov/pubmed/19715461

[190] "Formaldehyde in Your Home: What you need to know," Agency for Toxic Substances and Disease Registry.
https://www.atsdr.cdc.gov/formaldehyde/home/index.html

mizuna mustard, Red Russian kale and zinnia flowers, and envision future missions planting tomatoes, peppers, berries and beans."[191] And if NASA can grow plants in space without gravity, just think what you can do at home *with* gravity!

Convinced you don't have a green thumb? Frustrated with plants that do not live long, healthy lives indoors? Are you a victim of plant disasters? Don't worry, you can overcome these setbacks. They can generally be grouped into 3 categories.

First, sadly, many of the houseplants that are sold in supermarkets and mass retailers are doomed from the start. Their roots are aggressively hacked too short and/or the hacker has stuffed a large plant into a small pot. At the point of purchase, consumers may believe that they are getting a big plant for a small price, but it's just a doomed plant.

Second, too many plant owners let their plants get either too much or too little sun. The info-spikes that come with house plants usually have helpful suggestions, but sometimes they're dead wrong. For starters, experiment with indirect light. Most commonly sold house plants do well with indirect light, and may easily get fried with too much direct sunlight. In fact, a lot of house plants thrive with no direct sunlight at all. Pay attention when you bring home a new plant. Each plant needs housebreaking. It only takes a short while till you're both comfortable.

---

[191] Anna Heiney, editor, "Growing Plants in Space," National Aeronautics and Space Administration (NASA), Updated: Jan. 29, 2020.
https://www.nasa.gov/content/growing-plants-in-space

Third, many people overwater their plants, causing root rot and premature death. My mother taught me the solution to this. Just stick your finger in the soil. If it's moist, don't water the plant. If it's dry, add water. Pretty simple. And last but not least, some people just forget to water their plants. Again, this not complicated, after you water your plants, decide when they might need water again, and on the appointed date, write down on your calendar, "Plants." If one of your "Plants" watering days falls on a 6 month "25% LESS FRIES" or "25% LESS anything" party date, celebrate with your plants (just don't feed them cake). Your life will become *even more* exciting!

And now that you're an exhilarating, confident, year-round, indoor Earth Mother (or Father), remember that in 'The Big Salad' chapter with 'The Big Salad Dressing' recipe, it was emphatically stated, "Without fresh basil, your life will never be complete." Now, you can also guarantee your complete life by growing basil indoors. While it's a shame that many people fail at this elementary undertaking, a few simple tips can remedy this.

Basil grown outdoors can do very well with some, but not too much direct sun. Indoors, very little or no direct sun can work well. But if you want to max out your basil and allow a fair amount of direct sun, remember that they will need more water, and can easily be fried by the sun without enough watering.

Put your plants in a bright spot, and the most important thing to remember is: *never, never, never* water the soil directly. Gnats will move in, lay eggs, and kill your beloved basil plants. Top-watering your plants will attract them. If you have good drainage, and allow your plants to completely dry out, but not to the point of wilting, gnats' eggs and larvae will usually die in dry soil. Also, you absolutely need to do the following: before you housebreak and bond with your basil, check the bottom of the plastic pot holding your plant; if there are no finger-size holes with soil visible, take a sharp knife and gouge out 3 or 4 holes. Place the plant in a saucer or plastic dish, and only pour water into the dish, *never, never, never* into the soil. That's it. You'll have fresh basil when you want it, and your life will be complete.

For those seeking to attain true love or more herbal adventure,

*Are you going to Scarborough Fair?*
*Parsley, sage, rosemary, and thyme*
*Remember me to one who lives there*
*She once was a true love of mine*[192]

In Medieval times, herbs represented virtues. Parsley was comfort, sage was strength, rosemary was love, and thyme was courage. Basil has covered the broadest emotional landscape. For Hindus, basil (known as tulsi) represented love, eternal life and purification.[193] The Greeks and Romans associated basil with hatred and insanity. Then later on, basil became a symbol of love in Italy, and it has retained that meaning ever since. In Moldavian folklore, a young man who accepts basil from a young woman is destined to fall

---

[192] Simon and Garfunkel, "Parsley, Sage, Rosemary and Thyme." *Scarborough Fair/Canticle*, Columbia, 1966.

[193] Holly Beth Anderson, "Basil," HOLLYBETH ORGANICS, July 1, 2014. https://hollybethorganics.com/gardening/basil-2/

in love with her.[194] I guess I'm just insanely in love with basil (alas, somehow I lost track of the young woman who gave it to me, dammit). If your basil gets lonely, you can move in housemates parsley, sage, rosemary and thyme, as well as oregano and cilantro, who will get along happily right next to your basil pals.

[194] Amy Jeanroy, "8 Herbs That Symbolize Love and Romance," THE SPRUCE, Updated: Sept. 17, 2020. https://www.thespruce.com/herb-meanings-in-love-and-romance-1761964

# Notes Of Fruit

You certainly don't want to count yourself among the 90% of Americans who don't eat enough fruit.[195] And for those who love fruit, you may rest assured that consuming large quantities of fruit is fine as long as it's part of a balanced diet. However, a fruit-centric diet can cause problems. Steve Jobs famously often restricted himself primarily to fruit, on occasion eating just carrots and apples. His fascination with fruitarianism is in fact credited with inspiring his company's name. In his preparation to play Jobs in the 2013 movie JOBS, Ashton Kutcher tried adopting this diet, and wound up in the hospital with pancreatitis. Jobs died of pancreatic cancer in 2011, (but eating excessive amounts of fruit does not cause pancreatic cancer). Still, Kutcher got quite a scare. In his case and possibly Jobs, the lack of some necessary vitamins and minerals, and deficiencies of fats and proteins, are suspected culprits.[196]

---

[195] Seung Hee Lee-Kwan, lead author, "Disparities in State-Specific Adult Fruit and Vegetable Consumption-United States, 2015," CDC Morbidity and Mortality Weekly Report, Nov. 17, 2017.
https://www.cdc.gov/mmwr/volumes/66/wr/mm6645a1.htm?s_cid=mm6645a1_w&utm_source=STAT+Newsletters&utm_campaign=f26644060f-MR&utm_medium=email&utm_term=0_8cab1d7961-f26644060f-150444909

[196] Angela Haupt, "Ashton Kutcher's Fruitarian Diet: What Went Wrong?" U.S. NEWS AND WORLD REPORT, Feb. 7, 2013.

The main consideration with overeating fruit is its natural sugar. A lot of fruit equals a lot of sugar. The great advantage that whole fruit has is that it contains soluble and insoluble fiber, and together, these fibers prevent a lot of sugar from being absorbed too early in the digestive process.[197] But for many people, too much sugar and too much acid, even from fruit, can cause discomfort, bloating, reflux, heartburn, diarrhea and high blood sugar.[198] [199]

You probably have a bunch of favorite fruits. The ones that you like are hopefully the ones that like you. If you're looking for new fruit friends, the farms and gardens and produce markets have many to offer. Candidates for sampling abound. And don't forget the berries. Rich in antioxidants, fiber, vitamin C and manganese, berries help fight inflammation, can lower cholesterol, reduce cancer risk,

https://health.usnews.com/health-news/articles/2013/02/07/ashton-kutchers-fruitarian-diet-what-went-wrong

[197] Markham Heid, "Is It Possible to Eat Too Much Fruit?" TIME, June 6, 2018. https://time.com/5301984/can-you-eat-too-much-fruit/

[198] Lindsay Mack, "Yes, you can eat too much fruit-and it could be messing with your diet," INSIDER, Oct. 20, 2017. https://www.insider.com/eating-too-much-fruit-side-effects-2017-10

[199] Lily Nichols, "5 Signs You're Eating Too Much Fruit," LILY NICHOLS. https://lilynicholsrdn.com/5-signs-youre-eating-too-much-fruit/

promote heart health,[200] [201] brain health,[202] and can make any boring companion food burst with flavor. For quite a while, after giving up on blueberries because they didn't like me, I paid little attention to berries. Then I discovered that blackberries were my buddies. Strawberries are hugely popular, but as with many berries, strawberries are especially good at trapping and retaining pesticides. Organic berries are more expensive, but pesticide-free, and really much better alternatives.

Opinions of when you should and shouldn't eat fruit are abundant and contradictory. Eat fruits at breakfast, not at night. Eat fruits in between meals, but not with meals. Eat fruits at any time of the day. Eat fruits with vegetables. Eat fruits without vegetables. My suggestion is try all of the above and see how you feel. I don't think there is a universal plan that is perfect for everyone.

The one time I went on a cruise, 2 strong impressions were made. One, watching ravenous passengers stuff themselves 7 times a day was nauseating. And two, heaving up and down in the belly of an ocean-hurdling tin can was even more nauseating. Before I abandoned ship in Costa Rica, and vowed to never go near another

---

[200] Franziska Spritzler, "11 Reasons Why Berries Are Among the Healthiest Foods on Earth," HEALTHLINE, Updated: April 24, 2019. https://www.healthline.com/nutrition/11-reasons-to-eat-berries

[201] Arpita Basu, Michael Rhone, Timothy Lyons, "Berries: emerging impact on cardiovascular health," NUTRITION REVIEWS, Vol. 68, Issue 3, Mar. 1, 2010, pp. 168-177. https://www.ncbi.nlm.nih.gov/pmc/articles/PMC3068482/

[202] Elizabeth Devore, lead author, "Dietary intakes of berries and flavonoids in relation to cognitive decline," ANNALS OF NEUROLOGY, Apr. 26, 2012. https://www.ncbi.nlm.nih.gov/pmc/articles/PMC3582325/

floating bucket of bolts, I had dinner with the ship's doctor. When desserts were offered, he was the only one at the table who declined besides me. Since I was turning madras with queasiness, I knew why I passed, but I asked the good doctor why he skipped the big assortment. He said that one should never eat sugar right after a meal, even fruit. His advice was to wait at least 30 minutes, preferably an hour. He was thin and had a medical degree, and I was seasick and ready to jump overboard. The logic was good. Dumping a load of sugar on a full stomach is not a great idea. I adopted the plan, and it has worked for me ever since. I have found that eating fruits for breakfast, followed by spacing out 1 or 2 carb grazes, exercising late in the day on an empty stomach, and having my vegetables at dinner gives me maximum comfort, productive workouts, and the most sustained clear-headed thinking throughout the day. If your eating/digesting/working/exercising schedule is not altogether satisfying, try rearranging it. Eat different things at different times. See what it feels like. A new order may make a new you. Customize!

# Let's Get Nuts

*We're all excited*
*But we don't know why*
*Maybe it's 'cause*
*We're all gonna die*
*And when we do*
*What's it all for?*
*You better live now*
*Before the grim reaper come knocking at your door*
*Tell me, are we gonna let de-elevator bring us down?*
*Oh, no let's go!*
*Let's go crazy*
*Let's get nuts*[203]

Prince wrote LET'S GO CRAZY, and was praised for encouraging us to not allow "de-elevator" (Satan) to bring us down, and instead seek a higher power (God), but perhaps overlooked was the line, "Let's get nuts."

Botanically defined, most nuts are actually seeds. Almonds, brazil nuts, cashews, macadamias, pecans, pistachios, pine nuts and walnuts

---

[203] Prince, "Let's Go Crazy." *Purple Rain*, Warner Bros. Records, 1984.

are all seeds. This group of seeds are called tree nuts.[204] Peanuts are legumes. But since all of the above have similar nutrient profiles, they get called nuts by just about everyone.

Nuts and seeds are for everyone (even the faithless). Nuts are rich in minerals and healthy fats. But, "Let's go crazy" should not be applied to nuts only because they are very high in fat and calories. To be thin like Prince, handfuls of nuts are not recommended. At about 100 calories per handful,[205] it's very easy to overdo it.

For those who want to compare and contrast their nuts, one ounce, 28 grams of almonds clocks in at 161 calories, 14 grams of fat, 6 grams of protein, 3.5 grams of fiber, and boast high levels of vitamin E and magnesium. Almonds can reduce inflammation in people with type 2 diabetes,[206] and possess potential prebiotic properties.[207] Cashews are also high in magnesium, 1 ounce contains 155 calories, 12 grams of fat, 5 grams of protein and only 1 gram of fiber.

---

[204] Charlie Mellor, "What's the difference between nuts and seeds?" WOODLAND TRUST, Aug. 29, 2019. https://www.woodlandtrust.org.uk/blog/2019/08/difference-between-nuts-and-seeds/

[205] Christopher Wanjek, "What are Superfoods?" LIVE SCIENCE, Mar. 18, 2019. https://www.livescience.com/34693-superfoods.html

[206] Jen-Fang Liu, "The effect of almonds on inflammation and oxidative stress in Chinese patients with type 2 diabetes mellitus: a randomized crossover controlled feeding trial," EUROPEAN JOURNAL OF NUTRITION, June 22, 2012. https://www.ncbi.nlm.nih.gov/pubmed/22722891

[207] Zhibin Liu, lead author, "Prebiotic effects of almonds and almond skins on intestinal microbiota in healthy adult humans," ANAEROBE, Vol. 26, Apr. 2014, pp. 1-6. https://www.sciencedirect.com/science/article/abs/pii/S1075996413001935?via%3Dihub

Pistachios have a similar profile, 28 grams equals 156 calories, 12.5 grams of fat, 6 grams of protein, 3 grams of fiber, but are lower in magnesium. Walnuts are higher in calories (182) and fat (18 grams) and lower in protein (4 grams) and fiber (2 grams), but are a great source of the omega-3 fat alpha-linolenic acid (ALA), and have done well in studies showing decreased risk of cardiovascular disease,[208] and reducing inflammation.[209] Pecans contain polyphenols (which act as antioxidants), are high in calories (193) and fat (20 grams), lower in protein (3 grams), with fiber at 2.5 grams per ounce. Macadamias are high in calories (200) and fat 21 grams (but a good source of monosaturated fat),[210] low in protein (2 grams), fiber also at 2.5 grams. An ounce of Brazil nuts contains 182 calories, 18 grams of fat, 4 grams of protein and 2 grams of fiber; they are high in magnesium, and super high in selenium, which acts as powerful antioxidant that may reduce asthma symptoms and some cancers, protect against heart disease and mental decline, and can boost thyroid

[208] Deirdre Banel, Frank Hu, "Effects of walnut consumption on blood lipids and other cardiovascular risk factors: a meta-analysis and systematic review," AMERICAN JOURNAL OF CLINICAL NUTRITION, July, 2009, 90(1): pp. 56-63. https://www.ncbi.nlm.nih.gov/pmc/articles/PMC2696995/

[209] Yu-Lan Chiang, lead author, "The effect of dietary walnuts compared to fatty fish on eicosanoids, cytokines, soluble endothelial adhesion molecules and lymphocyte subsets: a randomized, controlled crossover trial, PROSTAGLANDINS LEUKOT ESSENT FATTY ACIDS, Oct.-Nov. 2012;87(4-5):111-7. https://www.ncbi.nlm.nih.gov/pubmed/22959886

[210] Ruairi Robertson, Ph.D., "What Are the Benefits of Monounsaturated Fats?" HEALTHLINE, Sept. 17, 2017. https://www.healthline.com/nutrition/monounsaturated-fats

health and immune function.[211]   A Brazilian study on brazil nuts found that LDL "bad" cholesterol levels were dramatically reduced with the ingestion of just four brazil nuts.[212]  It should be noted that quantities should always be kept low because consuming too many brazil nuts can cause selenium toxicity.[213]  One ounce of peanuts, the very popular legume, has 176 calories, 17 grams of fat, 4 grams of protein and 3 grams of fiber; and may help reduce risk factors for heart disease and diabetes,[214] however allergy to peanuts is among the most common food allergies found in children.[215]

Many people complain they don't like the taste of raw nuts, and prefer roasted nuts with added salt.  Generally, I've found that a lot of the raw, salt-free nuts you buy off the supermarket shelf or have delivered to your home are not fresh, and their staleness is the problem.  I would urge you to seek fresh, raw, organic, salt-free nuts. Find purveyors who can provide high-end, packed-fresh, crunchy

---

[211] Jillian Kubala, "7 Science-Based Health Benefits of Selenium," HEALTHLINE, Aug. 20, 2019.
https://www.healthline.com/nutrition/selenium-benefits#10

[212] Michael Greger and Gene Stone, *How Not to Die*. New York: Flatiron Books, 2017, pp. 26-27.

[213] Katherine Marengo, "What are the benefits of eating Brazil nuts?" MEDICAL NEWS TODAY, Apr. 17, 2019.
https://www.medicalnewstoday.com/articles/325000

[214] Ruairi Robertson, Ph.D., "The Top 9 Nuts to Eat for Better Health," HEALTHLINE, Sept. 26, 2018.  https://www.healthline.com/nutrition/9-healthy-nuts

[215] "Peanut Allergy," American College of Allergy, Asthma & Immunology, Updated: Mar. 14, 2019.  https://acaai.org/allergies/types/food-allergies/types-food-allergy/peanut-allergy

nuts, and you'll get great taste and superior nutrition. And to maintain freshness and taste, always keep them sealed tightly, in the refrigerator, the happy home to store all your nuts and seeds.

While a variety of nuts can maximize benefits, I have found that a small portion of one type of nut per day in a salad or as a snack is the most efficient, beneficial, easiest-to-digest, and weight-maintaining model for me. Almonds on Monday, pistachios on Tuesday, cashews on Wednesday, alternating nuts makes my life interesting, and gives me something to look forward to every day, (I know, sounds pathetic, I'm just nutty). Walnuts and pecans don't like me, and I don't like them, but the world is full of nuts, with many possible choices readily available. And since you may be cutting down on meat and fried foods, nuts are wonderful and nutritious replacements to improve your diet. Experiment with all sorts of nuts, give yourself options, customize!

## Seeds Are For The Birds

*I wanna fly like an eagle*
*To the sea*
*Fly like an eagle*
*Let my spirit carry me*
*I want to fly like an eagle*
*'Til I'm free*
*Oh, Lord through the revolution*[216]

Seeds are for the birds, and seeds are for humans too. If you want to fly like an eagle, soaring and diving, making hairpin turns and breathless aerial maneuvers, just eat a bunch of seeds (or join the Air Force). Actually, eagles eat mostly fish and a mix of small mammals like squirrels, prairie dogs, racoons and rabbits. What about starlings? They are amazing flyers. They eat some seeds, but also centipedes, spiders, moths and earthworms. I wish I could fly. Unfortunately, eating like a bird doesn't guarantee flying like one. I've observed birds eat lots of seeds and fly like, well, birds. I've also consumed mass quantities of seeds myself, and now when I leap into the air, I

---

[216] Steve Miller, "Fly Like An Eagle." *Fly Like An Eagle*, Capitol Records, 1976.

can sometimes reach an altitude of 10 inches, for flight times lasting as long as a fraction of a second.

Culinary seeds come from a variety of plant sources, including flowers such as sunflowers, vegetables like pumpkins, and crops developed for many other uses like flax and hemp. Calories average about 150 per ounce. Seeds provide excellent sources of healthy fats, fiber and protein. Flax seeds and chia seeds are fiber-rich, omega-3 fatty acid champs with two to three times the alpha-linolenic acid (ALA) of walnuts. The omega-3 fats in both of these seeds are found in their fibrous outer shells which are not easily digestible, so it's best to grind them before eating. Hemp seeds are one of the few plants that have all the essential amino acids that your body cannot produce, and lead the seed pack with 10 grams of protein per ounce; they are also high in magnesium, thiamine, zinc and polyunsaturated fats. Mustard seeds are a rich source of selenium, and have 7 grams of protein per ounce. Pumpkin seeds (aka pepitas) are rich in monounsaturated fats, magnesium, phosphorous, iron and zinc, and deliver 8 grams of protein per ounce. Sunflower seeds provide high levels of monounsaturated fats, can help reduce inflammation and cholesterol levels, and are very high in vitamin E.[217] [218]

At one time, many doctors believed that consuming seeds could cause diverticulitis, (an infection in the muscular wall of the colon),

[217] Heather Goesch, "9 Super Seeds Are Small but Mighty," FOOD & NUTRITION, July 1, 2016. https://foodandnutrition.org/july-august-2016/9-super-seeds-small-mighty/

[218] Ruairi Robertson, Ph.D., "6 Super Healthy Seeds You Should Eat," HEALTHLINE, Oct. 9, 2017. https://www.healthline.com/nutrition/6-healthiest-seeds

however, no link between eating seeds and diverticulitis has been proven. Seeds are high in fiber which is vital for gut health.[219] [220]

If you lower your sugar and salt intake even a little bit, your taste buds will become more sensitive and responsive to other flavors.[221] What may have been previously perceived as a bland-tasting seed can become a delicious treat bursting with flavor.

I can remember watching my favorite cartoons on television interspersed with an endless barrage of giddy, animated commercials, preying on children, extolling candy bars and sugary cereals, and now just thinking about them gives me a headache. My kernel-poor youth shall be redeemed by a seed-rich adulthood. As I gradually increased my nuts and seeds intake, without any additional exercise, I got thinner, and my cholesterol numbers improved. Whenever I have a bowl of grains, I look forward to topping it off with hemp hearts, ground flax and chia seeds. My favorite big salad is not complete without pumpkin and sunflower seeds. I love seeds, and they love me. Maybe one day, I'll be able to fly like an eagle, soar with the starlings, and leap *eleven* inches into the air.

---

[219] "Quick-start guide to nuts and seeds," HARVARD HEALTH LETTER, Sept. 2019. https://www.health.harvard.edu/staying-healthy/quick-start-guide-to-nuts-and-seeds

[220] "Diverticulitis," MAYO CLINIC, May 7, 2020. https://www.mayoclinic.org/diseases-conditions/diverticulitis/symptoms-causes/syc-20371758

[221] "Want to Cut Sugar, Salt, or Fat? Retrain Your Taste Buds," RALLY HEALTH, Aug. 2 2018. https://www.rallyhealth.com/weight/want-to-cut-sugar-salt-or-fat-retrain-your-taste-buds

# Part III: *Plants, Fish, Humpty Dumpty And Canned Spaghetti*

# A Fine Kettle Of Fish

Back in the meat chapters, we made the case for reducing or eliminating meat. And as we cut down on meat, we need good replacements. The benefits of the plant world are enormous, but satisfying all of our nutritional needs by relying solely on plants is challenging. Only a few protein-rich plants have all the necessary amino acids humans need, like our bud, the hemp seed.

And since our bodies can't make omega-3 fatty acids, fish should be a vital part of meal planning. Nuts, seeds and plant oils can provide adequate amounts of one of the key omega-3 fatty acids, namely, alpha-linolenic acid (ALA). But they lack the other two important omega-3s, docosahexaenoic acid (DHA) and eicosapentaenoic acid (EPA). Your body can convert some ALA into DHA and EPA, but only in tiny amounts. Consuming fish and other seafood is the only practical way to get DHA and EPA. Omega-3 supplements have not shown the same level of benefit.[222] A major study reported in the NEW ENGLAND JOURNAL OF MEDICINE found that omega-3 supplements did not reduce heart attacks, strokes, or deaths from heart

---

[222] "Omega-3 Supplements: In Depth," NIH National Center for Complementary and Integrative Health, Updated: May 2018. https://www.nccih.nih.gov/health/omega3-supplements-in-depth

disease.[223] [224] Salmon, herring and sardines have the highest levels of DHA and EPA. Mackerel, sea bass and trout are runners-up.[225]

Years ago, as I reduced meat consumption, I increased my seafood intake, eventually morphing into a pescatarian, or technically speaking, a lacto-ovo-pescatarian since I also eat eggs and dairy. Again, a gradual process of customizing myself over a period of time. If you want to go this route, try your own selection of fish and shellfish. See what you like and what likes you.

I stick with wild fish.

Wild fish swim greater distances and have a more varied diet than farm fish. Consider the good you garner with a diverse diet, and how wild fish may also achieve similar outcomes. Diversity promotes health and provides more sources of vitamins and minerals. Wild fish feed on smaller fish and tiny organisms like krill which eat algae, a rich source of omega-3 fatty acids. They are leaner, lower in fat and calories, darker in color, higher in protein, potassium, selenium, antioxidants and B vitamins, and usually higher in omega-3s, and lower in inflammatory omega-6s than farmed fish. Crowded conditions are the norm with farm fish which increases the risks of infection, and results in treatment with large doses of antibiotics. Wild fish come without added antibiotics. The pitch that farm-raised

---

[223] Howard LeWine, MD, "Fish oil: friend or foe?" HARVARD HEALTH PUBLISHING, Updated: Apr. 15, 2020.
https://www.health.harvard.edu/blog/fish-oil-friend-or-foe-201307126467

[224] "Omega-3 Fatty Acids," NIH Office of Dietary Supplements, Updated: Oct. 1, 2020. https://ods.od.nih.gov/factsheets/Omega3FattyAcids-Consumer/

[225] Ibid.

fish are more sustainable than wild fish does not hold water. It takes 2 to 3 pounds of often highly-processed, high-fat, fish feed concocted with a mix that may have genetically modified organisms (GMO) corn, grains and fish chow (other smaller fish) to make 1 pound of farm-raised salmon. Many varieties are higher in contaminants and cancer-causing chemicals like polychlorinated biphenyls (PCBs) and dioxin. Dyes are often added to gray-ish farm fish to make them look wild. (Coloring your hair is one thing, but coloring your fish?) And again, caveat emptor, pay attention to labels when shopping for fish. The moniker "Atlantic Salmon" is commonly applied to farm fish.[226] [227]

All of you avid label-readers should also keep an eye out for genetically engineered salmon. FDA-approved in 2019 as a "new animal drug," and dubbed "Frankenfish" by its detractors, this genetically altered *new salmon* is created by the insertion of a growth hormone gene from Chinook salmon into the genetic sequence of a typically less-traveled, farmed salmon. Doesn't that sound appetizing? And while manufacturers are required to disclose if their salmon is genetically modified, restaurants are exempt from revealing this to their customers.[228]

---

[226] David Perlmutter, MD, "5 Reasons Why You Should Avoid Farm-Raised Fish," davidperlmutter MD, May 21, 2014.
https://www.drperlmutter.com/5-reasons-avoid-farm-raised-fish/

[227] "Wild caught salmon vs farmed," Mind Over Munch.
https://mindovermunch.com/blog/wild-caught-salmon-vs-farm-raised/

[228] Michelle Pugle, "Would You Eat Genetically Modified Salmon?" HEALTHLINE, June 29, 2019. https://www.healthline.com/health-news/would-you-eat-genetically-modified-salmon

And as long as we're on the subject of restaurants, there are way too few in the USA that are really good at providing a wide array of fresh, expertly-prepared, wild seafood. If you can find one, be a good customer. The same goes for markets. All the fish you see behind the glass should look mahvelous, dahling. If it doesn't look fresh, it ain't fresh.

Another sad reality is that seafood is often mislabeled, which is a charitable way of saying, the claim is wild, but the reality is farm-raised. Oceana did a fascinating study, using DNA testing, collecting 82 salmon samples from restaurants and grocery stores to determine that 43% were mislabeled, most of which, 69% were actually farmed salmon being sold as wild-caught. The study found this practice everywhere it tested: 48% in Virginia, 45% in Washington, D.C., 38% in Chicago and 37% in New York.[229] Consider your sources. It's worth the effort to find the most reliable ones. Catching your own is a pretty good idea too. We've all heard, 'Give a man a fish, and you feed him for a day. Teach a man to fish, and you feed him for a lifetime.' Our guide, Lao-tzu has been credited with this proverb.[230] Since he so kindly articulated the first step of our journey, we should again be grateful.

It's no mystery that many people who don't like fish were soured by a single bad experience. One serving of rank, over-the-hill, *fishy*

---

[229] Kimberly Warner, Ph.D., "Oceana Reveals Mislabeling of American's Favorite Fish: Salmon," OCEANA, Oct. 2015.
https://usa.oceana.org/publications/reports/oceana-reveals-mislabeling-americas-favorite-fish-salmon

[230] Anne Isabel Thackery Ritchie, QUOTE INVESTIGATOR, Aug. 28, 2015.
https://quoteinvestigator.com/2015/08/28/fish/

fish is often enough to make a person swear off fish forever. Granted, it's gross, but you can have the same bad luck with milk, eggs, meat or any other food that should have been thrown out before it got near a consumer.

Wild salmon is one of the greatest sources of nutrition in the world. Ask any bear who resides near a river in The Great Northwest. If you happen to not love salmon, it may be because you have not experienced the tremendous variety of flavors that can range from delicate to robust, and not *fishy*. Try to find a fish market that has many varieties of wild salmon. The one I go to has 6 on a good day. They can be grilled, steamed, baked or poached, yielding all sorts of gustatory reactions. Try medium or well done to further alter or refine the taste. Raw salmon sushi or sashimi reveal another, distinctive spectrum. Sample an inexpensive can of skinless and boneless wild salmon to get the same nutritional benefits with a milder taste. Put it in a salad, or mix it with mayonnaise, and compare it to your favorite tuna and mayonnaise combo. You may prefer the salmon as I do.

It's remarkable that so many fish have survived the human abuses of overfishing and industrial pollution. The aquatic ecosystem has been challenged by the toxic effects of heavy metals in particular. Mercury, cadmium, copper, aluminum, chromium, lead and zinc are the main pollutants, posing danger for the fish exposed to them and the humans who consume these fish.[231] In general, the larger and older the fish, the higher the level of heavy metal contamination.

---

[231] Mohammad Authman, lead author, "Use of Fish as Bio-indicator of the Effects of Heavy Metals Pollution," JOURNAL OF AQUACULTURE, Vol. 6, Issue 4, 2015. https://www.longdom.org/open-access/use-of-fish-as-bioindicator-of-the-effects-of-heavy-metals-pollution-2155-9546-1000328.pdf

Location, diet and habitat are also factors. Some big fish at the top of the ocean food chain that should be limited or avoided include: swordfish, king mackerel, tilefish, barramundi, orange roughy, albacore, yellowfin and bluefin tuna. Lower on the food chain, smaller, safer, better choices include: salmon, skipjack tuna (chunk light), snapper, whiting, sardines, anchovies, perch, cod, calamari, and shellfish like shrimp, lobsters and oysters.[232]

Harvard School of Public Health professors Dariush Mozaffarian and Eric Rimm have done extensive work on the effects of toxins in the oceans, concluding that the benefits of eating fish far outweigh the risks of heavy metal pollution.[233]  Considering polychlorinated biphenyls (PCBs) pollution, (typically higher in farm fish), from Environmental Protection Agency (EPA) data and elsewhere, they calculated that if 100,000 people ate farmed salmon for 70 years, the extra PCB intake might cause 24 extra cancer deaths, but would prevent at least 7,000 deaths from heart disease.  Other studies point out that while high intake of mercury appears to hamper a baby's brain development, low intake of omega-3 fats from fish is at least as dangerous.  In a LANCET study of nearly 12,000 pregnant women, children born to those who ate less than 2 servings of fish per week did worse on tests of intelligence, behavior and development as

---

[232] Naturopath, "Heavy Metals in Fish," Superpharmacy, Dec. 3, 2017.
https://www.superpharmacy.com.au/blog/heavy-metals-in-fish

[233] Dariush Mozaffarian, Eric Rimm, "Fish intake, contaminants, and human health: evaluating the risks and the benefits," JAMA, Oct. 18, 2006;296(15):1885-99.
https://jamanetwork.com/journals/jama/fullarticle/203640

children from mothers who ate fish at least twice a week.[234] Pregnant women should keep in mind that avoiding seafood completely is likely to harm their babies' brain development.[235] Swimming with the little fish is the best way to travel.

Several canned tuna sellers have made efforts to offer products with lower mercury levels. Wild Planet tries to limit mercury content by sticking with younger, lighter fish (9 to 25 pounds) which are naturally lower in mercury.[236] Safe Catch has a proprietary tool which takes a small sample from a fish, and analyzes the mercury content. Fish with low percentages are purchased. Fish with higher percentages are not. Safe Catch CEO Sean Wittenberg claims, "Our mercury standards are 70% below the FDA's mercury limit for albacore, and 90% below their limit for skipjack tuna."[237]

As with finfish, shellfish provide high quality sources of protein. All of the essential amino acids reside under their armor. A 3 ounce serving delivers the same amount of protein as an equal portion of

---

[234] Joseph Hibbein, lead author, "Maternal seafood consumption in pregnancy and neurodevelopmental outcomes in childhood (ALSPAC study): an observational cohort study," LANCET, Feb. 17, 2007;(9561):578-85. https://www.thelancet.com/journals/lancet/article/PIIS0140-6736(07)60277-3/fulltext

[235] "Fish: Friend or Foe?" Harvard T.H. Chan School of Public Health, The Nutrition Source, https://www.hsph.harvard.edu/nutritionsource/fish/#1

[236] "The Wild Planet Tuna Procurement Policy," Wild Planet Foods, Updated: Feb. 2017. https://wildplanetfoods.com/wp-content/uploads/2018/10/Wild-Planet-Procurement-Policy-2.2017_FINAL.pdf

[237] Stephanie Eckelkamp, "The New Way To Buy Mercury-Free Canned Tuna," PREVENTION, Dec. 31, 2014. https://www.prevention.com/food-nutrition/healthy-eating/a20429219/mercury-free-tuna-from-safe-catch/

90% lean ground beef. Saturated fat levels are a tiny fraction of those found in meat. Crabs, clams, crayfish, lobster, scallops and shrimp have 2-5% of the saturated fat as lean ground beef. Shellfish are also good sources of omega-3 fatty acids. Mussels and oysters are especially high in omega-3s. Beef has zero.[238]    Important micronutrients like selenium, iodine, iron, copper, zinc and vitamin B12 abound in shellfish.[239]    For fun and nutrition, decapitate a decapod, and bash some shells!

Granted, seafood consumption presents challenges regarding freshness, purity, preparation and sustainability, but in comparison to the resource-depleting, climate-degrading, virus-promoting, worker-mistreating, hormones/pesticides/antibiotics-adding practices of factory meat production, I say, Go Fish!

---

[238] "Heart Beat: Shellfish for the Heart?" HARVARD HEART LETTER, Dec. 2009. https://www.health.harvard.edu/newsletter_article/shellfish-for-the-heart

[239] Faye M. Dong, "The Nutritional Value of Shellfish," Washington Sea Grant, University of Washington, Revised: 2009. https://wsg.washington.edu/wordpress/wp-content/uploads/publications/Nutritional-Value-of-Shellfish.pdf

# Canned Spaghetti And The Sardine Principle (Plus Tips On Surviving Pandemics, Biological Warfare, Terrorism, Nuclear Winters, Climate Disasters, Earthquakes, Camping Trips, And How To Make Food Taste Better)

Sardines are a fantastic source of nutrition. A 4.25 ounce tin of Atlantic Ocean sardines contains 170 calories, 22 grams of protein, 9 grams of fat, and no starch or sugar. Sardines provide excellent sources of omega-3 fatty acids, vitamins B2, B3, B12 (super-high levels) and D, selenium, phosphorus, calcium, copper and choline. Residing ultra-low on the food chain, consuming mainly plankton, sardines have insignificant amounts of mercury and other contaminants.[240]

An adorable little fish, an athletic swimmer, and oh boy, are they good for you!

But who loves sardines?

Most people don't love sardines, including me. But applying the wild salmon approach of trying all the variations and preparations imaginable, I have found that it is possible to customize and elevate

---

[240] "Sardines" Precision Nutrition,
https://www.precisionnutrition.com/encyclopedia/food/sardines

the sardine experience to an enjoyable level. First off, skip the sardines packed in soybean oil, and avoid sardines in packed olive oil. Soybean oil is high in omega-6 fatty acids which offsets the benefit of eating omega-3 rich sardines in the first place.[241] And, some of the nutrients in sardines can leach into olive oil, the excess of which you drain off. Also, the olive oil used to pack sardines is generally of a low or mediocre quality, with much poorer taste than a topnotch extra virgin olive oil (EVOO). This can be critical because the not-so-terrific flavor of sardines is a challenge to begin with. Adding anything not-too-wonderful is not recommended. A well-stocked market will offer dozens of brands and varieties. I suggest hunting down a wild-caught, no-salt added, skinless, boneless, packed in-water variety. If the flavor is still too strong for you, try refrigerator-chilling first, then drain, and spread out on a plate. Fresh squeezed lemon is optional, but it can take the edge off. Now, cover the fillets with your finest EVOO and a mountain of fresh basil. And when I say mountain, I mean mountain. You need a healthy pile of fresh basil to compete with, tame, and best case scenario, enhance the strong taste of sardines.

Admittedly, still not my favorite dinner, but somehow, sardines possess a special, magical power. Along with super-nutrition, they provide a valuable counterpoint and contrast to whatever upcoming

---

[241] Karen Collins, "Sardines in oil don't always have good omegas," THE SAN DIEGO UNION-TRIBUNE, Nov. 18, 2007.
https://www.sandiegouniontribune.com/sdut-sardines-in-oil-dont-always-have-good-omegas-2007nov18-story.html

gastronomic experience may be in store for the adventurous consumer. Perhaps these little fish deliver a kind of unconscious anticipation of something better. It could be a secret ability to set in motion a delayed sensory reaction. I have discovered that whatever I eat the next day tastes incredible! I could eat a tennis shoe, and WOW, it's delicious!

I make it my business to eat sardines once a week. Twice a week, no thanks. But once a week works fine. It's sort of like camping. If you've ever camped out, you know that just about anything you eat tastes *way better* outdoors in the glow of a campfire, even a can of spaghetti.[242]

---

[242] Sardine tins stack easily, and keep fresh for a long time. A tall stack will last longer than a short stack, and come in handy when facing the next pandemic, climate disaster, earthquake, act of war or other unwelcome event.

# The Best Meal I Ever Had

*So if you are the big tree*
*We are the small axe*
*Ready to cut you down (well sharp)*
*To cut you down*[243]

Without a doubt, the best meal I ever had in my whole life was when I was a Boy Scout, stalwart member of BSA Troop 4, Panther Patrol, Tuscan School, Maplewood, New Jersey, USA. We were a small troop, a motley crew, but dedicated to learning new skills, assuming meaningful responsibilities, and being good Scouts. As far as I know, we had the good fortune to be free from the horde of child molesters who posed as scoutmasters, and are now being outed by the tens of thousands. For me and my friends, it was an innocent time.

Somehow, I was appointed Troop Scribe. I didn't ask for the job. I was anointed. My writing career was launched. I had a weekly column in the local paper, NEWS-RECORD OF MAPLEWOOD AND SOUTH ORANGE. I got to wear an embossed patch with 2 crossed quill pens on my left sleeve right below the troop numeral. The new Boy Scouts of America Scribe patch has only 1 quill. What

[243] Bob Marley, "Small Axe." *Burnin',* Island-Tuff Gong. 1973.

happened to the other quill, I don't know. The Boy Scout motto is 'Be Prepared.' It's a great motto. I've tried to live by it my whole life.

For me and most of my cohorts, the greatest feature of scouting was camping. And as fate would have it, one of Troop 4's most arduous camping trips planted the seed for 'Canned Spaghetti And The Sardine Principle.'

It was the middle of the winter, snow was in the forecast, and while some of the parents were skeptical of having their suburban children lugging massive knapsacks, hiking straight uphill to South Mountain Reservation, pitching tents, chopping wood, building fires and sleeping outside in the freezing cold, we fearless, intrepid Scouts of Panther Patrol were totally psyched. Eventually, all of the parents realized that getting a bunch of hormonally challenged, obnoxious 12 year olds out of the house for a few days made a lot of sense, so we were all approved for The Trip.

Embracing the Be Prepared motto, I had everything planned perfectly except for a couple of special requirements that needed to be met in order to Be *Totally* Prepared for The Trip.

One, I had to convince my mother that I absolutely, positively could not survive in the freezing woods of South Mountain Reservation in the middle of winter without my very own Boy Scouts of America official, regulation hatchet. An ample supply of wood would need to be chopped, hauled and fed to a roaring fire in order to prevent certain death. Somehow, she bought it. I was so stoked! Getting that killer axe was life-changing. My confidence soared! Nothing could stop me now. Thor just had a hammer. I had an axe! An official, regulation BSA fire engine red axe, and thick leather

185

sheath with slits for my official, regulation BSA belt to go through and hug that awesome weapon to my hip. Not exactly Wyatt Earp's Colt .45, but pretty close. I wish I had that hatchet today. I don't know what I'd do with it, but I wish I had it now.

Two, I knew that a long, cold day of hiking, tent-pitching, wood-chopping, and fire-feeding would require a hot meal for dinner. But how much dinner stuff could I fit into an overstuffed knapsack that already weighed almost as much as I did? This might be an even bigger challenge because the utterly elegant solution I came up with was the acquisition of a single can of spaghetti. Simple, right? Not with my mother. The idea of her child eating spaghetti out of a *can* was unthinkable. I begged and argued, even suggesting that I might have to hunt down a squirrel or a snake, and kill it with my hatchet, and maybe get bitten by a wild animal and die, but no, no way, no *can* of spaghetti would ever enter her home, even to be hustled out the door in my knapsack.

The solution turned out to be a contract, a solemn oath, that I would never eat spaghetti out of a can for the rest of my life *if* she granted me an exception just this one time. And it worked! I'd worn her down. She bought a can of spaghetti with my father's hard earned cash. We both vowed to keep a secret.

And so, I was Prepared. I and my troop marched uphill all day to reach our destination. I chopped armloads of vital fuel for our life-saving campfire. Exhausted and starving, I heated up that can of spaghetti in the roaring fire, managing somehow to not burn myself, and deliriously wolfed down 1 full can of mushy spaghetti suspended in red stuff that was alleged to be tomato sauce.

Now at this point, you may be thinking, so what? Who in their right mind would get excited about eating a can of spaghetti? Under normal circumstances, no one. But, under extreme circumstances, in the freezing cold, leaning into a blazing fire, ravenous, I experienced a can of spaghetti that was beyond ambrosial. My taste buds have never exploded like that. It was, and still is, the tastiest, best meal I've ever had! (If you need more evidence, check out THE SOPRANOS episode, "Pine Barrens," and watch the reactions of lost/freezing/starving Christopher and Paulie when they consume a couple of ketchup packets).[244]

Acquiring the hatchet was the peak of my scouting career. I had intended to one day make Eagle Scout, but the little axe convinced me that I didn't need the Scouts anymore. I got what I came for. If I wanted to, I could kill a charging buffalo with that hatchet. Axe in hand, I knew I was Prepared for life beyond scouting.

But the can of spaghetti taught me a greater lesson. You can actually control the taste of food. You don't need massive amounts of sugar to excite your taste buds. Your enjoyment of food can be affected by a variety of environmental and psychological factors. If you alter your circumstances, you can change, improve and customize your diet.

Canned spaghetti is not the greatest choice for nutrition, but lending my experience with 1 can of spaghetti to countless tins of

---

[244] THE SOPRANOS, season 3, episode 11, "Pine Barrens." Written by Terrence Winter and Tim Van Patten; directed by Steve Buscemi; Christopher (Michael Imperioli), Paulie (Tony Sirico), HBO, May 6, 2001. Chosen by TV GUIDE as the fourth-best episode of the 21st Century. Video: https://www.youtube.com/watch?v=pOYKTjXY1EQ

sardines has benefitted me greatly. Try this at home. Apply 'Canned Spaghetti And The Sardine Principle' to a food that you're not crazy about, but you know is good for you. Pay attention to how your taste buds react the next day. It's a new sensation! (Also confirmed by INXS).

*Live baby live*
*Now that the day is over*
*I gotta new sensation*
*In perfect moments*
*Well so impossible to refuse…*
*…Gotta hold on you*
*A new sensation, a new sensation*
*Right now gonna take you over*
*A new sensation, a new sensation*
*-INXS* [245]

[245] Andrew Farriss, Michael Hutchence, INXS "New Sensation," *Kick*, WEA-Atlantic-Mercury, 1987. Video:
https://www.youtube.com/watch?v=azfG5H-pCVg

# The Lobster Principle

'The Lobster Principle' is the harmonizing inverse of the 'The Sardine Principal.'

You can demonstrate this concept with your favorite, special dinner. (If you're not sure what your favorite special dinner entrée is, just ask yourself what you'd request for your last meal if you were about to be executed. That's it. That's your special dinner).

In my case, it's lobster. Canadian lobsters are OK, Maine lobsters are better, but New Jersey lobsters are the best. (I can already hear people in New England screaming at me). Maine lobsters are sweet. New Jersey lobsters are brinier. It's a subtle difference. I really like Maine lobsters, but I prefer the briny snap of a Jersey lobster.

After more than 50 years of fervent investigation, I have concluded that the best way to achieve the most intensely scrumptious, satisfying lobster experience is to schedule the lobsters at least seven days apart. So, theoretically, to attain the highest number of profoundly joyful lobster meals in a given year, that would allow for an annual maximum of 52 lobsters, spaced exactly seven days apart, for 52 weeks in a row. This may be anecdotal evidence, but it has withstood the test of time for over 5 decades of blissful shellfish ingestion.

Have you ever had lobster 2 days in a row? Seems excessive, doesn't it? A little over the top? A double dose of evening cholesterol, make that a quadruple dose if you add melted butter.

On several occasions, during my early lobster-scheduling research, for the sake of science, I ate lobster 2 days a row. I no longer do this for a variety of practical and health reasons, but I couldn't help noticing, in every case, the lobster I ate the second day didn't taste as good as the one from the day before. It didn't feel as good going down. I didn't get the same rush, the just-right, full-body satisfaction, the Zen-like afterglow. Maybe it was some kind of gut guilt, perhaps it was my gut telling me that once a week is enough, that two in a row is too much, or hey, give me a break, I'm still recovering from last night. Maybe lobster likes me, but it doesn't like me *that* much.

The point here is, you can feel better, and gain greater enjoyment from your favorite foods if you don't overdo it. This theory works with all sorts of foods. You can find this feel better/enjoy-it-more activity apparent with proteins, fats and carbs. It works with Jersey lobsters, Georgia peaches and chocolate cupcakes (but take it easy on the cupcakes).

Try eating sardines for dinner 1 night, then the next night, have a lobster. It will blow your mind!

# Slam Dunk Fish Stew

For anyone leery about enjoying, prepping, cooking or cleaning up a fish mess, 'Slam Dunk Fish Stew' is my highly-evolved, fast-and-easy, lean-and-not-mean, skip-the-butter-and-cream, nutritious-and-delicious, fish-and-vegetable stew for the CUSTOMIZE YOURSELF generation. I've added, subtracted, changed and customized this recipe many times over many years. You can do the same. Below is my latest iteration.

*SLAM DUNK FISH STEW (Serves 4)*
*Extra virgin olive oil (EVOO) (2-3 tablespoons, or substitute with an equal amount of 'The Big Salad Dressing')*
*Cod (1.5 pounds)*
*Pepper (1 large orange or yellow)*
*Mushrooms (2 large, or 4 small)*
*Tomato (1 medium or large Jersey tomato or Heirloom variety, or 2 plum tomatoes, or 6 Campari tomatoes)*
*Sweet potato (1 medium purple or 2$^{nd}$ choice, orange)*
*Oregano (8-10 fresh leaves, or 2-3 pinches of dry oregano)*
*Garlic (1 minced garlic clove, or a pinch of dry garlic)*
*Turmeric (2-3 pinches)*
*Basil (16-24 fresh leaves)*

*Arugula (16-24 fresh leaves)*
*Fresh ground black pepper to taste*
*Salt to taste*
*Water (12 ounces)*

**1)** Cut tomato, pepper and mushrooms into small to medium chunks. Cut sweet potato into slices or chunks.

**2)** Using a thick-bottom, 2.5 quarts or larger pot, pour EVOO or 'The Big Salad Dressing' into the pot, and swirl around to cover the sides.

**3)** Cut cod into large chunks and put in pot, or just layer in the whole fillet(s).

**4)** Pile in vegetables, herbs and spices (but *not* the basil or arugula) on top of the fish. Put the sweet potato in last.

**5)** Pour in 12 ounces of water.

**6)** Bring to a boil, then maintain a low boil for 30 minutes, or until fish is cooked through and easily flakes apart.

**7)** Ladle into 4 bowls or plates. Let cool for a few minutes, then cover with arugula and basil leaves, and serve.

If you're dining solo, ladle 1 portion into a bowl or plate for yourself, then put the other 3 portions in small bowls, let cool, cover with plastic wrap, put in plastic bags, and freeze. For a future quick dinner, you can defrost a bowl, heat/microwave and eat PDQ, no fuss, no muss, no bother.

## Humpty Dumpty Got A Raw Deal

*Humpty Dumpty sat on a wall,*
*Humpty Dumpty had a great fall;*
*All the king's horses and all the king's men*
*Couldn't put Humpty together again.*[246]

Many historians have asserted that Humpty Dumpty was a large cannon used by the British Royalists to fend off the Parliament's army during the English Civil War. After the Parliamentary artillery damaged the wall beneath Humpty Dumpty in 1648, well, Humpty fell. However, even before then, in 15th century England, Humpty Dumpty was a common nickname for overweight people. Others have claimed that Humpty Dumpty was King Charles I, or King Richard III, or Cardinal Wolsey from the Henry VIII era.[247] [248]

---

[246] Mother Goose.

[247] "The Egg-Citing Truth Behind Humpty Dumpty," RIPLEY'S BELIEVE IT OR NOT!, July 4, 2019. https://www.ripleys.com/weird-news/humpty-dumpty/

[248] "Humpty Dumpty and the Fall of Colchester," MYTHS AND LEGENDS, 2006. http://myths.e2bn.org/mythsandlegends/origins1-humpty-dumpty-and-the-fall-of-colchester.html

So how did Humpty Dumpty become an egg? In 1871, Lewis Carroll's THROUGH THE LOOKING GLASS depicted Humpty as a large egg with eyes, nose and mouth, arms and legs, dressed in pants and shoes (unlike Donald Duck), perched on a wall, just another wise guy conveniently located to annoy a passing girl. And this disagreeable, anthropomorphic egg has since inspired many tales of suspicion and consternation involving eggs. (Besides promoting nutritious carrots, even Bugs Bunny was once conned by the Easter Bunny to deliver eggs for him, only to face more shotgun blasts from Elmer Fudd.)[249]

Western nutritionists used to regularly bash eggs as high cholesterol, heart-attacking, little bombs that were unhealthy and should be avoided. At the dawn of the 21st century, the American Heart Association advocated a cholesterol limit of 300 milligrams per day.[250] More recently, they published a torturously worded advisory stating that, "Evidence from observational studies conducted in several countries generally does not indicate a significant association with cardiovascular disease risk."[251] Either eggs hired a new publicist or they evolved from shell-delivered killers into a new "superfood." Among the most nutrient-dense foods on earth, one large egg contains 6 grams of protein with all the essential amino

---

[249] *Easter Yeggs*, Warner Bros. 1947.

[250] Ronald Krauss, lead author, "Circulation," American Heart Association, Oct. 31, 2000.
https://www.ahajournals.org/doi/10.1161/CIR.0000000000000743

[251] Jo Ann Carson, lead author, "Dietary Cholesterol and Cardiovascular Risk: A Science Advisory From the America Heart Association," Dec. 16, 2019.
https://www.ahajournals.org/doi/10.1161/CIR.0000000000000743

acids, only 77 calories, 5 grams of healthy fats, and significant amounts of vitamins A, B2, B5, B6, B12, folate, choline, phosphorus, selenium and zinc.[252]

At 212 milligrams, eggs are indeed high in cholesterol, but this does not necessarily raise cholesterol in the blood. Every day, a healthy liver produces large amounts of cholesterol. As you consume more dietary cholesterol, your liver produces less.[253] In 70% of people, eggs don't raise cholesterol at all. In the other 30%, eggs can mildly raise total and LDL (bad) cholesterol, but the overall effect is positive. This is related to the fact that LDL particles are divided into two types: 'small,' dense LDL particles, and 'large' LDL particles. While many studies have concluded that people who have mostly 'small' LDL particles have a higher risk of heart disease,[254] egg consumption appears to change the pattern of from 'small' LDL to 'large' LDL which is linked to a reduced risk of heart disease.[255] Also, eggs raise HDL (good) cholesterol. While diabetics are advised

[252] "Egg, whole, cooked, hard-boiled Nutrition Facts & Calories," SELF, 2018. https://nutritiondata.self.com/facts/dairy-and-egg-products/117/2

[253] Maria Luz Fernandez, "Dietary cholesterol provided by eggs and plasma lipoproteins in healthy populations," CURRENT OPINION IN CLINICAL NUTRITION AND METABOLIC CARE, Feb. 2006. https://www.ncbi.nlm.nih.gov/pubmed/16340654

[254] C.D. Gardner, lead author, "Association of small low-density lipoprotein particles with the incidence of coronary artery disease in men and women," JAMA, Sept. 18, 1996;276(11):875-81. https://www.ncbi.nlm.nih.gov/pubmed/8782636

[255] Kris Gunnars, "Top 10 Health Benefits of Eating Eggs," HEALTHLINE, June 28, 2018. https://www.healthline.com/nutrition/10-proven-health-benefits-of-eggs#section5

to discuss eating eggs with their doctors, multiple studies have found that egg consumption by people without diabetic issues is not associated with increased risk of coronary heart disease or stroke.[256] [257]

One egg contains 150 milligrams of choline, a vital nutrient that many people don't get enough of. Egg yolks have one of the most concentrated source of choline available. Choline-deficiency has been cited as having an impact on liver disease, atherosclerosis, breast cancer risk, and some neurological disorders. Studies showing that fetuses consume 6 to 7 times as much choline as adults have induced doctors to advise pregnant and lactating women to increase their intake of choline.[258] [259] [260]

---

[256] Ying Rong, lead author, "Egg consumption and risk of coronary heart disease and stroke: dose-response meta-analysis of prospective cohort studies," BMJ, Jan. 7, 2013;346:e8539. https://www.ncbi.nlm.nih.gov/pmc/articles/PMC3538567/

[257] William Boden, "High-density lipoprotein cholesterol as an independent risk factor in cardiovascular disease: Assessing the from Framingham to the Veterans Affairs High—Density Lipoprotein Intervention Trial," THE AMERICAN JOURNAL OF CARDIOLOGY, Nov. 30, 2000, 86(12A):19L-22L. http://europepmc.org/article/MED/11374850

[258] Emily Boynton, "Nutrient in Eggs and Meat May Influence Gene Expression from Infancy to Adulthood," University of Rochester Medical Center, Sept. 20, 2012. https://www.urmc.rochester.edu/news/story/3617/nutrient-in-eggs-and-meat-may-influence-gene-expression-from-infancy-to-adulthood.aspx

[259] Jian Yan, lead author, "Pregnancy alters choline dynamics: results of a randomized trial using stable isotope methodology in pregnant and nonpregnant women," AMERICAN JOURNAL OF CLINICAL NUTRITION, Dec. 2013; 98(6): 1459-1467. https://www.ncbi.nlm.nih.gov/pubmed/24132975

[260] Steven Zeisel, Kerry-Ann da Costa, "Choline: an essential nutrient for public health," NUTRITION REVIEWS, Vol. 67, Issue 11, Nov. 2009, pp. 615-623. https://www.ncbi.nlm.nih.gov/pmc/articles/PMC2782876/#R11

Egg yolks also contain large concentrations of lutein and zeaxanthin, potent antioxidants that accumulate in the retina of the eye. Consuming these nutrients can significantly reduce the risks of cataracts and macular degeneration.[261] [262]

Hens who are allowed to roam in the sunshine and/or receive omega-3 enriched feeds, produce eggs with additional nutritional benefits. Higher in vitamin D and omega-3s, these eggs can significantly lower triglycerides.[263]

[261] Richard Roberts, lead author, "Lutein and zeaxanthin in eye and skin health," CLINICS IN DERMATOLOGY, Vol. 27, Issue 2, March-April 2009, pp. 195-201.
https://www.sciencedirect.com/science/article/abs/pii/S0738081X08000126

[262] Cecile Delcourt, lead author, "Plasma Lutein and Zeaxanthin and Other Carotenoids as Modifiable Risk Factors for Age-Related Maculopathy and Cataract: The POLA Study," INVESTIGATIVE OPTHALMOLOGY & VISUAL SCIENCE, June 2006, Vol. 47, Issue 6.
https://iovs.arvojournals.org/article.aspx?articleid=2125160

[263] Pascal Bovet, lead author, "Decrease in blood triglycerides associated with the consumption of eggs of hens fed with supplemented with fish oil," NUTRITION, METABOLISM AND CARDIOVASCULAR DISEASES, Vol. 17, Issue 4, June 28, 2006, pp. 280-287.
https://www.sciencedirect.com/science/article/abs/pii/S0939475306000214

While published studies about eggs may continue to report conflicting results, many have gone so far to declare that eating up to three eggs per day is completely safe.[264] [265]

And so Humpty Dumpty is back up on the wall, defending British royalty, or harassing young girls, or waiting for a frying pan. I have been thriving on 2 eggs every other day for a long time. I look for 'USDA Organic' and 'Free Range' on the carton. Let's hope Humpty doesn't have another great fall.

---

[264] Kris Gunnars, "Top 10 Health Benefits of Eating Eggs," HEALTHLINE, June 28, 2018. https://www.healthline.com/nutrition/10-proven-health-benefits-of-eggs

[265] Kris Gunnars, "Eggs and Cholesterol – How Many Eggs Can You Safely Eat?" HEALTHLINE, Aug. 23, 2018. https://www.healthline.com/nutrition/how-many-eggs-should-you-eat

## Gut Check

Probiotics are beneficial bacteria that naturally live in your body, keep it healthy, balanced and functioning well. They also fight off bad bacteria, help your body digest food, create vitamins, and support cells that line your gut to prevent bad bacteria from entering your blood. Probiotics are an integral part of your microbiome, a unique collection of trillions of microbes combining bacteria, fungi, viruses and protozoa.[266]

A key word here is *unique*. Endless claims are made by purveyors and consumers of probiotic supplements as to what is best for everybody. The flies in their ointments are stuck in the conundrums of what is best for everybody is different for everybody, and, there are no reliable, proven plans to *customize* for anybody.

Do you have any probiotics-obsessed friends who are convinced that you should consume the probiotics supplements they tout? I have a few. They mean well, but would probably be better served by eating a variety of foods rich in probiotics. Fermented foods like cottage cheese, kimchi, sauerkraut, pickles, yogurt (some Greek yogurt has added probiotics like lactobacillus acidophilus and lactobacillus

---

[266] "Probiotics," Cleveland Clinic, 2020.
https://my.clevelandclinic.org/health/articles/14598-probiotics

casei), miso and kambucha are rich in probiotics.[267] You may not like every one of these foods, and they may not like you, so if you're game, try one at a time, gauge your reaction, and strive to customize.

If your supplement-taking friends proselytize or get annoying, try pointing out that the probiotics supplement industry resembles an unregulated, amorphous echo chamber designed to sell products (with the more syllables, the better). Most probiotics are sold as dietary supplements which do not undergo the tests and approvals required for drugs.[268] And even though probiotics should contain live cultures, there's no guarantee that the bottles deliver what's printed on the label.[269]

For more aggravation, you can find hundreds of websites pointing out why you should avoid all the probiotics in the world except the ones they are promoting and selling. Claims and accusations regarding quality, effectiveness, sources, purity, handling, freshness, refrigeration, additives, dosages, expiration dates, packaging and advertising are designed to direct consumers to their products and the phenomenal benefits only they can provide. They quote studies, often small, short duration, inconclusive, or non-human/animal-based, and extrapolate fantastic associations between the data and their products.

---

[267] Alexandra Sifferlin, "10 Foods Filled With Probiotics," TIME, Apr. 12, 2018. https://time.com/5236659/best-probiotic-foods/

[268] "Health benefits of taking probiotics," HARVARD HEALTH PUBLISHING, Updated: Apr. 13, 2020. https://www.health.harvard.edu/vitamins-and-supplements/health-benefits-of-taking-probiotics

[269] Amanda Macmillan, "Here's Everything You Need to Know About Gut Health," TIME, Updated: Apr. 1, 2019. https://time.com/5556071/gut-health-diet/

And they have demonstrated some extraordinary sales to back their hype. Global probiotic sales were pegged at over $48 billion in 2018,[270] and projected to exceed $64 billion by 2023.[271]

But what do the scientists who are not reaping huge profits from selling probiotics have to say?

Dr. Gail Hecht, chair of the American Gastoenterological Association for Gut Microbiome Research and Education notes, "A lot of probiotic strains are not what you would naturally find in large quantities in the human intestine. So you can eat them or drink them, but they won't necessarily do you any good."[272]

Krzysztof Czaja, associate professor of veterinary biosciences at the University of Georgia points out that trying to figure out which foods or probiotics could possibly harmonize the microbiome and improve health is like baking a perfect cake with 5,000 different ingredients, "The idea that eating this fruit or popping that supplement will do the trick is a woeful oversimplification of the microbiome's complex role in human health. If your goal is to encourage healthy

---

[270] "Probiotics Market Size, Share & Trends Analysis Report By Product (Food & Beverages, Dietary Supplements), By Ingredient (Bacteria, Yeast), By End Use, By Distribution Channel, And Segment Forecasts, 2019 – 2025," Grand View Research, June, 2019. https://www.grandviewresearch.com/industry-analysis/probiotics-market

[271] Gregor Reid, lead author, "Probiotics: Reiterating What They Are and What They Are Not," FRONTIERS IN MICROBIOLOGY, Mar. 12, 2019; 10: 424. https://www.ncbi.nlm.nih.gov/pmc/articles/PMC6425910/

[272] Amanda Macmillan, "Here's Everything You Need to Know About Gut Health," TIME, Updated Apr. 1, 2019. https://time.com/5556071/gut-health-diet/

gut bacteria communities, there is no perfect food or perfect bacteria cocktail."

And Dr. Vincent Young, professor of microbiology and immunology at the University of Michigan Medical School adds, "We're still learning what is a 'healthy' microbiome. There's tremendous promise, and the research is being done, but right now, we don't know what's deranged or lacking, or how to fix it. You will always have unexpected side effects, some of which you can't predict when manipulating a complex system."[273] [274]

Plenty of claims have been made that probiotics may be useful in treating certain medical conditions like diarrhea, constipation, inflammatory bowel disease (IBD), irritable bowel syndrome (IBS), yeast infections, urinary tract infections, gum disease, lactose intolerance, eczema, sepsis and upper respiratory infections. But results can vary greatly, and what works for one person may not work for another.[275] A 2020 report from the American Gastroenterological Association (AGA) says that probiotics don't do much for gut health, including conditions like Crohn's disease, ulcerative colitis or irritable bowel syndrome. "For the majority of the digestive diseases

---

[273] Markham Heid, "It's Not Yet Clear How to Boost the Microbiome. But Diet Is the Best Bet," TIME, Aug. 8, 2018. https://time.com/5360407/microbiome-diet-gut-health/

[274] Saman Khalesi, lead author, "A review of probiotic supplementation in healthy adults: helpful or hype?" EUROPEAN JOURNAL OF CLINICAL NUTRITION, Mar. 26, 2018. https://www.nature.com/articles/s41430-018-0135-9

[275] "Probiotics," Cleveland Clinic, 2020. https://my.clevelandclinic.org/health/articles/14598-probiotics

we studied, currently there is not enough evidence to recommend using probiotics," according to Dr. Geoffrey Preidis, a pediatric gastroenterologist at the Texas Medical Center and spokesperson for the AGA. He also notes that probiotics may be harmful in some circumstances, "Among the more serious side effects is infection. As living microbes, probiotics can leave the intestines and enter the bloodstream, causing sepsis."[276] Before attempting to treat any medical condition with probiotics, you should check with your doctor.

*Pre*biotics are a type of fiber that your body cannot digest, and serve as food for probiotics. There is less research and compelling data on prebiotics than on probiotics. Plunging into prebiotic supplements is at least as murky a venture. The good news is that prebiotics occur naturally in many foods.[277] Garlic, onions, leeks, asparagus, bananas, barley, oats, apples, cocoa, chickpeas, artichokes and flaxseed are all good sources of prebiotics.[278] Pick out the ones that you like, stick with the ones that like you, and customize!

If you lie awake at night wondering what new tools may be deployed to launch targeted attacks on specific bacteria, upcoming research may show how to effectively use CRISPR (Clustered

---

[276] Katie Hunt, "Probiotics don't do much for most people's gut health despite the hype, review finds," CNN HEALTH, June 9, 2020. https://www.cnn.com/2020/06/09/health/probiotics-new-us-guidelines-wellness/index.html

[277] Zawn Villines, "What is the difference between prebiotics and probiotics?" MEDICAL NEWS TODAY, Oct. 29, 2018. https://www.medicalnewstoday.com/articles/323490

[278] Arlene Semeco, "The 19 Best Prebiotic Foods You Should Eat," HEALTHLINE, June 8, 2016. https://www.healthline.com/nutrition/19-best-prebiotic-foods

Regularly Interspaced Short Palindromic Repeats) to alter the human microbiome in specific, personalized ways from person to person. According to David Edgell, Ph.D., Professor, Schulich School of Medicine & Dentistry, University of Western Ontario, "Using CRISPR to kill things isn't a new idea… The problem has always been how you get CRISPR to where you want it to go. Other delivery systems could only go to a few spots, where ours can go anywhere."[279] As Amazon and Walmart have figured out better ways to deliver pickles and yogurt to your front door, advanced CRISPR targeting may one day provide a more customized tool for your gut. Stay tuned.

While the scientists are constructing further studies, feed your mysterious probiotics with some enigmatic prebiotics. You should be able to come up with a better plan for your unique microbiome than an overzealous supplement maven marketing microbe merchandise.

---

[279] Crystal MacKay, "Researchers unlock potential to use CRISPR to alter the microbiome," PHYS.ORG, Oct. 4, 2019. https://phys.org/news/2019-10-potential-crispr-microbiome.html

## True Hydration

Are you losing electrolytes? Do you know where to find them? Have you checked in the Lost and Found? Have you been convinced by the sports drink industry that they can replace your lost electrolytes (for a small charge)? Would you recognize an electrolyte if you met one in a bar? What's all the fuss about electrolytes?

Electrolytes are essential minerals that conduct electricity when mixed with water. They regulate hydration, blood, nerve and muscle function, and are a part of the tissue rebuilding process. You may not find them in the Lost and Found, but your body needs all of them, namely: sodium, calcium, potassium, magnesium, bicarbonate, chloride and phosphate. And they have to be in the right balance. Too much or too little can result in numbness, weakness, exhaustion, headache, nausea, muscle spasm, blood pressure changes, bone or nervous system disorders, irregular heartbeat, confusion, seizures or feeling just plain lousy.[280]

Electrolyte levels change when water levels change. Excessive sweating, alcohol consumption, vomiting or diarrhea may cause rapid

---

[280] Adam Felman, "Everything you need to know about electrolytes," MEDICAL NEWS TODAY, Nov. 20, 2017.
https://www.medicalnewstoday.com/articles/153188

changes. It's important to be hydrated and stay hydrated after exercise. Don't let bottled water marketing lead you to drink more water than you need. Drink too much water and you lose sodium.

The author of AGE LATER, Dr. Nir Barzilai, founding director of the Institute For Aging Research at Albert Einstein College of Medicine, and a leader in advancing the science of longevity, says that men need at least 4 cups of water per day, and women need 3. These amounts can rise with exercise, higher altitudes, lower humidity, and higher temperatures.[281]

Dr. Christian Gonzalez, a Naturopathic Doctor who specializes in Integrative Oncology, is the host of HEAL THY SELF, a mega informative podcast that covers a wide range of topics relating to health and healing. For an excellent 2 hour primer on hydration, podcast episodes #61 and #82,[282] including insights from hydration educator and consultant Tracy Duhs, take a deep dive into water, water, water. Regarding water consumption, Dr. Gonzalez advocates drinking half your body weight in ounces per day. But, drinking water out of plastic bottles is not recommended. Besides our monstrous, plastics pollution problems, plastic bottles leak bisphenol A (BPA), a chemical that disrupts our hormones, inflames our brains and messes with our immune systems.[283] And to muddy the water some more,

---

[281] Nir Barzilai, *Age Later.* New York: St. Martin's Press, 2020.

[282] Christian Gonzalez (Dr. G), HEAL THY SELF podcasts #61 and #82 can be found here: https://podcasts.apple.com/us/podcast/heal-thy-self-with-dr-g/id1455361893

[283] Jenny Carwile, lead author, "Polycarbonate Bottle Use and Urinary Bisphenol A Concentrations," ENVIRONMENTAL HEALTH PERSPECTIVES, Sept. 1, 2009, Vol. 117, No. 9, pp. 1368-1372. https://www.ncbi.nlm.nih.gov/pmc/articles/PMC2737011/

plastic bottles stamped with 'BPA Free' may be even more toxic. Studies have shown that BPA substitutes like bisphenol S (BPS) have similar or worse effects than BPA.[284]

If you're hooked on bottled water, pay attention to independent test results, presence of electrolytes, and protection levels of their sources. And for Mother Earth's sake, be sure to recycle.

Perhaps Elon Musk or Jeff Bezos could take a break from racing to Mars, and find a safe and human/planet-healthy alternative to the ubiquitous plastic bottle? If you know a rich person looking to improve life on Earth, go ahead, twist their arm. According to FORBES,[285] there are at least 2,095 billionaires in the world. How about one of you guys pitching in to make a better bottle? Find a chemical engineer who can solve it, license it, make a few more billion, and move up on the FORBES list. Slow Death By Chemical Leaching Plastic Bottle is not as dramatic as Life Or Death On Mars, but really, now, here, on the planet we *need* to save, let's focus our attention. Earthlings unite!

Tap water in America is also in a sorry state. Lots of improvement needed here. Contaminated drinking water can lead to birth defects, developmental delays in children, gastrointestinal disease,

---

[284] Eric Stann, "Think all BPA-free products are safe? Not so fast, scientists warn," SHOW ME MIZZOU UNIVERSITY OF MISSOURI, release, Feb. 18, 2020. https://showme.missouri.edu/2020/think-all-bpa-free-products-are-safe-not-so-fast-scientists-warn/ and "Warning Signs: How Safe Is BPA Free?" ENDOCRINE NEWS, Aug. 2016. https://endocrinenews.endocrine.org/warning-signs-how-safe-is-bpa-free/

[285] As of Mar. 18, 2020, FORBES lists 2,095 billionaires. https://www.forbes.com/billionaires/

neurological disease, hormonal disruption, immune disfunction and cancer. Lead pollution is still a problem in many locations. Perfluoroalkyl substances (PFAS), like Teflon and Scotchgard, also known as "forever chemicals" because they don't break down, are linked to cancer and other maladies. In 2018, the EPA estimated that 110,000,000 Americans may be contaminated with PFAS. Since then, findings by the Environmental Working Group (EWG) say the number may be much higher.[286] The EPA says PFAS should not exceed 70 parts per trillion. The EWG sets a safety limit of 1 part per trillion. Quite a gap!

Water quality in the cities and towns of America varies greatly. To check on yours, go to EWG's Tap Water Database: https://www.ewg.org/tapwater/ Type in your zip code to get the number of contaminants that exceed EWG health guidelines in your area. Your local water company is required to regularly test your water, and publish reports. It's worth your time to read these reports.

Water filters can make a big difference. Dr. Gonzalez has analyzed many of them, and has decided to use the Travel Berkey Water Filter, priced at $249. If you're on a budget, Dr. G recommends the Propur G 2.0, which as of this writing was listed on Amazon for $52.46.

His podcast guest, Tracy Duhs has studied the effects of combining clean water with trace elements. She emphasizes that that these minerals are needed to get water into your cells. Achieving the right

---

[286] Sydney Evans, lead author, "PFAS Contamination of Drinking Water Far More Prevalent Than Previously Reported," ewg.org, Jan. 22, 2020. http://www.ewg.org/research/national-pfas-testing/

balance will determine how much water you need. Tracy adds that, 'True Hydration' needs to be supported with all sorts of movement, play, (including grown-up adults bouncing on trampolines), grounding and sunshine. A sandy beach helps. San Diego-based Tracy is living proof. Her HYDRATE PODCAST[287] will inform your water molecules. Since 98.9% of your molecules are water molecules, you have plenty to enlighten. She is the Queen of Hydration.

Applying the above along with your CUSTOMIZE YOURSELF skills, you can fine tune your water consumption, and avoid dehydration. Strive to get all the electrolytes you need with a well-balanced, well-customized diet. Fruits and vegetables are excellent sources of electrolytes.

We'll get deeper into hydration in CUSTOMIZE YOURSELF: FITNESS, but for now, if you're exercising moderately, for up to 60 minutes, you're probably OK with just drinking water. With heavier or more intense exercise, don't forget your friend, the banana, or perhaps consider a sports drink or a bottled water that's electrolyte-rich or has added electrolytes. But if you're going the sports drink route, check the ingredients. Many have too much added sugar and food coloring, or may not have enough electrolytes to resupply your body after a heavy workout.[288]

---

[287] HYDRATE PODCAST With Tracy Duhs can be found here: https://tracyduhs.com/podcasts/

[288] Kyle Beswick, "What are Electrolytes?" CEDARS-SINAI BLOG, Oct. 16, 2019. https://www.cedars-sinai.org/blog/electrolytes.html

Optimum hydration can provide health and healing. Headache relief and better sleep are yours for the drinking. Manage your hydration to enhance energy, mental acuity, and joint fluidity. Stay moist, my friends!

# Eating In The 21st Century

Way back before digital video recorders, Facebook, Google, YouTube, Twitter, Instagram, TikTok and Russian KGB/GRU/FSB/IRA operations and trolls[289] ran the United States, the American zeitgeist was crafted by Mad men, aka Madison Avenue advertising executives, like the men in hats brought to life in the TV series MAD MEN.[290] In those pre-DVR days, everybody had to watch all the commercials. Americans paid close attention, and bought the beer, soda, cigarettes and highly processed food products which formed many of the habits still widely practiced today in nutritionally-challenged America. Handed down from generation to generation, product-driven eating practices established in the dawn of television in the 1950s and 60s, still prevail in many 21st century households. If we could undo even a fraction of the brainwashing of

---

[289] Just a few of the Russian (previously Soviet) intelligence agencies/operations engaged in security functions and projects like destroying democracy and running the world: Komitet Gosudarstvennoy Bezopasnosti (KGB) or "Committee for State Security," Glavnoya Razvedyvatel'noye Upravleniye (GRU) or "Main Intelligence Directorate," Federal'naya Sluzhba Bezopasnosti (FSB) or "Federal Security Service," and The Internet Research Agency (IRA) or fondly known in Russia as the "Trolls from Olgino."

[290]*Mad Men*, Lionsgate Television, 2007-2015.

America, we'd all be healthier, but since that's not possible, we should at least pay attention to how profoundly we are manipulated by marketing and propaganda.

The CUSTOMIZE YOURSELF approach is helpful in this regard, and the 'More Harm Than Good' list you so assiduously compiled at the end of that chapter is also a good tool. So let's go back, and give your list a tune-up. If you haven't at least knocked off 25% of your grease and sugar intake, do it now. You'll feel really silly in 6 months without something to celebrate. And who wants to go through life in an unenviable state of physical and mental decline as a mere pawn of the commercial puppet masters who only want you alive so they can sell you their products?

One of the less obvious messages of early TV advertising was the notion that more is better. And lots more is lots better. "Betcha can't eat just one!" was Lay's Potato Chips slogan for decades. And they were right. It was a clever challenge to hook customers who then went overboard eating chips. This phenomenon was identified as "hedonic hyperphagia," by Dr. Tobias Hoch and his team at FAU Erlangen-Nuremberg in Erlangen, Germany. They pioneered in using magnetic resonance imaging (MRI) to observe rats' brains light up like Times Square when they were fed potato chips vs. another group of rats who only received boring rat chow.[291]

Comedic deployment of foods as props was also a popular vehicle to sell things. One of the longest running comedies in Broadway

---

[291] "Revealing the scientific secrets of why people can't stop after eating one potato chip," American Chemical Society, Apr. 11, 2013. https://www.eurekalert.org/pub_releases/2013-04/acs-rts030713.php

history was GEMINI, launched in 1976, and propelled by a hit TV commercial with a mother yelling at her son stuffing his face, "Take human bites!" and, a woman leaning into her boyfriend's plate with, "I'm not hungry, I'll just pick," and sucking up a plateful of spaghetti.[292]  It was fun to eat like a character on TV, so America laughed and gobbled right along with their televisions.

My family gobbled right along with the rest of America, and I was the biggest gobbler of all.  My dear mother's lightning reflexes were honed daily every time she put a plate of food on the table.  She had to recoil in a flash to avoid being stabbed by a piercing volley of forks bayonetting everything in sight.  I don't know why eating became attacking, but it did.  I didn't mind eating like a dog.  I admired dogs because they could eat so fast, even faster than I could, not much faster, but definitely faster.  Freed from the awkward manipulations of knives, forks and spoons, dogs gleefully just dive right in. Occasionally, when I was closing in on dog-eating velocity, my mother would blurt out, "You'd think someone is trying to take it away from you!"  At some point, when I was aggressively shoveling it in, my brother Marc said, "One day we'll be here eating meat and potatoes and you'll be eating salads!"  Well, he was right about that, but at the time, the mere suggestion of missing out on future meat and potatoes-binging gave me pause.  Maybe I should slow down?  Was it even possible?  The funny thing was, while I was attacking food like the Tasmanian Devil, (the one in the Warner Bros. cartoons, not a real Tasmanian devil), my sister Joan was being mocked by my

---

[292] GEMINI Broadway commercial with Danny Aiello, video:
https://www.youtube.com/watch?v=Pz8p6-LconE

brother because she ate so slowly. She explained that she took a course in school that conveyed the benefits of eating slowly, and was fully committed to it. We watched her eat slowly like it was something strange and unnatural. Like an exotic creature who somehow wound up at our dinner table. She finished every meal 20 minutes after the rest of us. Even my mother and father thought that was unusual. And it kind of gave me cover for my extreme habits. Years later, when I embraced the slower-is-better method, I gradually decelerated/customized to an easygoing pace that allowed me to savor and enjoy my food, to eat less and benefit more. Now I finish 20 minutes after Joan.

Eating fast is just a habit. Watching television is also a habit. Eating fast and watching television is a habit that encourages the consumption of too many calories, gaining weight, and enjoying food less. When I was progressively slowing down my madcap masticating, I was lucky enough to get the helpful expression stuck in my head, EAT TO LIVE, DON'T LIVE TO EAT. It still pops up in my brain, and I pay attention. Benjamin Franklin is credited with coining this. He became a vegetarian at age 16 to save money and buy more books,[293] but a savory Atlantic cod (see 'Slam Dunk Fish Stew') convinced him to add fish to his diet.[294] For most of his adult life, at 5'9" and 220 pounds, he struggled with obesity, but lived to

---

[293] *The Autobiography of Benjamin Franklin.* London: J. Parson's, 1793.

[294] Ibid.

age 84,[295] pretty impressive for those days.  He was a nation's savior, and maybe a cod was his savior.  Just a guess.  For Ben's sake and your own, go back to your 'More Harm Than Good' list, and print at the bottom in big capital letters, EAT TO LIVE, DON'T LIVE TO EAT.

And while you're at it, leave some space to write, PORTION CONTROL, PORTION CONTROL, PORTION CONTROL.  (If you're a real estate agent, look at the spot where you have tattooed "Location, Location, Location" and add, "Portion Control, Portion Control, Portion Control").

Trade in your big plates for smaller plates.  Figure out how much food you want on your plate, put exactly that amount on the plate, then put everything away.  Don't leave any other plate, bowl, bag, box or package of food open and sitting on a counter for easy access, instead wrap up everything and put it away, then place your plate on the table, and enjoy!  Make believe you're in a restaurant.  When you're in a restaurant, you can't get up, walk into the kitchen and pile more food on your plate.  (It's frowned upon.  And if you've ever worked in a restaurant, you know that there are some chefs who'll grab their biggest knife, and chase you the hell out of there).  At home, like in a restaurant, eat the food on your plate, and you're done.  Stop eating.  Leave the table.  Sit in an easy chair.  Read a book.  Watch TV.  Sing.  Dance.  Walk the dog.  Do the laundry.  If you don't have a dog, you probably have laundry.  The point is, you decide how much

---

[295] "Benjamin Franklin," notednames.com, https://notednames.com/Politician/American-Politician/Benjamin-Franklin-Birthday-Real-Name-Age-Weight-Height/

to eat ahead of time, rely on your good judgement, and follow your custom plan.

If you're hell-bent on dessert, wait at least 30 minutes. Whether it's fruit (fructose) or a cookie (refined sugars), you don't want to dump a load of sugar on top of your carefully planned meal. Give your gut some to time to digest, and make room for more food rather than just expand more and more, and be burdened by an unnecessary sugar load. Again, *portion control, portion control, portion control.* Don't snuggle up to a bagful of cookies on your cushy sofa, and gorge. Remove 1 cookie, put it on a plate or napkin, close up the bag, and put it away, then sit down, get comfortable, and slowly savor the cookie. Consider dessert as a reward. If you get too many rewards for doing basically nothing, the rewards become meaningless. You carry your excessive rewards around in your gut and they become an unhealthy, unsightly burden. If you even think about getting up for another cookie, remember 'The 10 Minute Rule.' Just wait 10 minutes. After 10 minutes, you won't even be hungry.

If you're in a situation with other diners, and there's a gleaming, frosted cake or a stack of thick, chewy brownies staring at you, there's no point in torturing yourself. Call, "Time out!" and go to a neutral corner. Think of it like a boxing match. You just knocked out your opponent, and the referee sends you to your corner while he counts to ten.

Your very personal, gradually-developed, logically-evolved, carefully-honed,
steadily-improved, time-tested, confidence-building, *unique*, custom plan has been created for you, by you, and nobody else. You didn't suffer with some diet guru until you hated their regimen. *You* made a

better life for yourself. And you will continue to refine, extend and enjoy your eating escapades to make your life the best it can be. You are in control of your destiny. You will be healthier, happier and more vital than you ever imagined as you continue your journey of a lifetime to CUSTOMIZE YOURSELF!

# About the Author

Chuck Rose has spent most of the last 50 years customizing, evolving a set of simple, useful techniques to improve and integrate nutrition, fitness and mindbody connection, growing from an overweight kid mesmerized by ecstatic cartoon characters raving about the euphoria of sugar, into a lean, athletic adult who no longer quotes Tony the Tiger.

In between pandemics, Rose also devotes time to exploring the art of cinema. As founder, curator and moderator of Arthouse Film Festival (AFF), he has informed and entertained live audiences for 29 years, interviewing 1,194 filmmakers and actors for AFF while also producing and moderating post-screening discussions and seminars for Paramount, Universal and SAG-AFTRA Foundation.

Spending time on both coasts, Rose has authored 30 screenplays, directed VIETNAM VETS starring Danny Aiello, worked in the story department at Orion Pictures, served as a Contributing Editor at MOVIES USA and written feature articles on the film industry for THE HOLLYWOOD REPORTER.

He has held faculty positions at Seton Hall University, Adelphi University and The New School for Social Research. Rose is an alumnus of the Warner Bros. Writers Workshop, and holds an MA from the University of Southern California and a BFA from New York University.

His greatest joy is swimming in the Atlantic Ocean, or the Pacific, or whatever ocean is convenient. While his 10 sitting-on-the-edge-of-the-planet summers as a lifeguard in Pt. Pleasant Beach, New Jersey are fading into history, he promises to stay fit enough to help out on a rough day.

www.customizeyourself.org

Made in the USA
Middletown, DE
11 November 2021